Junietta Baker McCall, DMin

Grief Education
for Caregivers
of the Elderly

*Pre-publication
REVIEWS,
COMMENTARIES,
EVALUATIONS . . .*

"**T**his book gives us a succinct, yet elegant, presentation of the problems encountered in helping elderly people face death, grief, and bereavement. It is a thoughtful and compassionate book that is based on the author's extensive experience as a chaplain at New Hampshire Hospital, a public psychiatric hospital. Much of her work consists of pastoral care for elderly residents of the hospital's psychiatric nursing home.

There are excellent chapters on the phenomenology of grief and bereavement that encompass with empathy the perspective of older persons, including the grief of growing old itself. Prejudicial views of older people are effectively challenged by Dr. McCall.

The chapter about clergy as caregivers is especially insightful and gives the reader an implicit awareness of the author's own spirituality.

The book's purpose is to educate people who care for those who are old and ill about grief, in both themselves and in their patients. It succeeds admirably. It will be of help and of interest to all who work to enhance the lives of older people."

Richard B. Ferrell, MD
*Associate Professor of Psychiatry,
Dartmouth Medical School,
Hanover, NH*

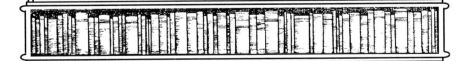

"**A**n old Spanish proverb says, 'It is not the same to talk of bulls as to be in the bullring.' This book is written from the vantage point of the author who has spent her time in the 'bullring' of grief education. The ideas are honed on the anvil of her personal experiences with grief, in grief education, and being with dying persons and their survivors. June McCall has written a sound personal and professional volume that thoroughly integrates theory and practice in grief education.

In addition to thoughtful ideas about grief and grief education, the author has many excellent diagrams, outlines for workshops on different topics in the field, sensitive poems, and moving examples to flesh out the key ideas. To prepare oneself to be up to date in grief education, this book is must reading. I particularly like the chapters on the caregivers and the clergy as caregivers, in which she challenges them to become 'recovered healers' to those wounded by loss and grief."

Merle R. Jordan, ThD
Professor Emeritus
of Pastoral Psychology,
Boston University
School of Theology

"**T**his is more than a 'how to' manual. The author gets in touch with the assumptions, beliefs, and values of the caregiver in the context of everyone having a story that is a 'treasure to be shared.' She movingly describes the journey of elders toward death as a developmental life journey. She challenges caregivers (hospital staff, counselors, clergy) to involve themselves in grief education and she provides a very clear model developed in the hospital setting in which she works. The model includes the importance of understanding the needs of elders in the dying process. Dr. McCall moves Henri Nouwen's image of the 'Wounded Healer' to the 'Recovered Healer' who is present to the personal wounds of grief and loss in the life journey. Caring for the elderly dying person inescapably requires the authentic use of self. McCall captures this compellingly when she states that 'today we speak of eldercare as caring for others, but we know, deep inside us, that tomorrow eldercare is about caring for ourselves.'"

Marygrace McCullough, Dmin
Co-Director,
Interfaith Counseling Service,
West Newton, MA

"**T**his book is a thorough review of many theories and perspectives on aging, grief, and grief therapy. This will be helpful to all persons working in these fields. The chapter on 'Clergy As Caregivers' will be especially helpful to clergy in defining the problems they face and in helping them to set goals and objectives for working with elders, the bereaved, and the dying. The chapter on 'Envisioning Eldercare: The Next Fifty Years' is particularly stimulating as our culture prepares for the aging of the baby boom generation. Overall, I found this to be a careful study of major issues I face as a minister, a pastoral counselor, and a chaplain, and will recommend the book for use in our clinical pastoral education programs."

Richard B. Haines, DMin
Department of Chaplaincy Services and Pastoral Education, University of Virginia Health System

The Haworth Pastoral Press
An Imprint of The Haworth Press, Inc.

Grief Education
for Caregivers
of the Elderly

THE HAWORTH PASTORAL PRESS
Religion and Mental Health
Harold G. Koenig, MD
Senior Editor

New, Recent, and Forthcoming Titles:

A Gospel for the Mature Years: Finding Fulfillment by Knowing and Using Your Gifts by Harold Koenig, Tracy Lamar, and Betty Lamar

Is Religion Good for Your Health? The Effects of Religion on Physical and Mental Health by Harold Koenig

Adventures in Senior Living: Learning How to Make Retirement Meaningful and Enjoyable by J. Lawrence Driskill

Dying, Grieving, Faith, and Family: A Pastoral Care Approach by George W. Bowman

The Pastoral Care of Depression: A Guidebook by Binford W. Gilbert

Understanding Clergy Misconduct in Religious Systems: Scapegoating, Family Secrets, and the Abuse of Power by Candace R. Benyei

What the Dying Teach Us: Lessons on Living by Samuel Lee Oliver

The Pastor's Family: The Challenges of Family Life and Pastoral Responsibilities by Daniel L. Langford

Grief Education for Caregivers of the Elderly by Junietta Baker McCall

Somebody's Knocking at Your Door: AIDS and the African-American Church by Ronald Jeffrey Weatherford and Carole Boston Weatherford

Grief Education for Caregivers of the Elderly

Junietta Baker McCall, DMin

The Haworth Pastoral Press
An Imprint of The Haworth Press, Inc.
New York • London

Published by

The Haworth Pastoral Press, an imprint of The Haworth Press, Inc., 10 Alice Street, Binghamton, NY 13904-1580

Cover design by Monica L. Seifert.

Library of Congress Cataloging-in-Publication Data

McCall, Junietta Baker.
    Grief education for caregivers of the elderly / Junietta Baker McCall.
        p.   cm.
    Includes bibliographical references and index.
    ISBN 0-7890-0498-4 (alk. paper).
    1. Bereavement in old age. 2. Grief. 3. Loss (Psychology) in old age. 4. Death—Psychological aspects. 5. Care of the sick. 6. Caregivers. I. Title.
BF724.85.G73M33   1999
259'.6'0846—dc21   98-28105
                                                                                          CIP

This book is dedicated to my father, Cecil,
who taught me to be curious;
to my bright and gifted mother, Eleanor;
and to Aunt JoAnn.

ABOUT THE AUTHOR

Junietta Baker McCall, DMin, is Director of Pastoral Services at New Hampshire Hospital in Concord. Her previous positions include teaching in the Chicago Public School System, where she worked with developmentally challenged children, and Associate Pastor of South Congregational Church of Concord. An ordained minister of the United Church of Christ, Dr. McCall serves as adjunct faculty in pastoral counseling at Andover Newton Theological School in Newton Centre, Massachusetts. In addition, she is a Diplomate in the American Association of Pastoral Counselors, Director of Training at Journeys Pastoral Counseling Center in Durham, New Hampshire, and a Board-Certified Pastoral Counselor.

CONTENTS

Acknowledgments

I am grateful to all those who have helped and supported me in this endeavor. I am especially thankful for my husband, John Pearson. His quiet support, expressive encouragement, and confidence have helped me to complete this work. I am also grateful for my sons, who have filled my life with joy and encouraged me when I felt "stuck" at the computer. It was Seth who taught me about turning tough projects into successful products, and it was Jeremiah who encouraged me to write and who became a helpful technical resource.

I am fortunate to be working at New Hampshire Hospital where there is a commitment to grief education and quality care for patients, residents, and staff. I extend special thanks to the staff and residents of the Psychiatric Nursing Home. This work could not have been completed without the input, support, and shared leadership of Harry Woodley, who has been a valued colleague for many years. In addition, I want to express my deep appreciation to J. Earl Thompson Jr. for his guidance, and the sharing of his experience in the field of grief and loss.

To friends, relatives, colleagues, patients, and residents, some very much alive and many who are leading a gentle life somewhere in the wind—thank you.

Introduction

On his eightieth birthday John Quincy Adams responded to a query concerning his well-being by saying: "John Quincy Adams is well. But the house in which he lives at present is becoming dilapidated. It is tottering upon its foundation. Time and the seasons have nearly destroyed it. Its roof is pretty well worn out. Its walls are much shattered and it trembles with every wind. I think John Quincy Adams will have to move out of it soon. But he himself is quite well, quite well." (DeMoss and DeMoss, 1974, p. 13)

AN OLD WOMAN'S STORY

Sarah was born toward the tail end of the nineteenth century. She was bright and fairly good-looking and attended school with the children in her neighborhood. She read well and enjoyed reading at school programs and in her local church. She also sang and played music. In fact, she found much comfort in both words and music. She loved to have people around her. When I met her, she was in a nursing home and the mother of a now middle-aged child. She had many physically complex and challenging ailments and also suffered from depression. She had lived over half of her life away from home and had in fact come to call this nursing home her "home." Through her ninety-fifth year, she read and sang, worked with thread and needle, and greeted visitors. She dressed up for parties and looked forward to personal visits. On her birthday, she would say to me, "I'm just eighteen!" In her ninety-sixth year she became ill. It was difficult for her to breathe. We thought she would not live long. After a particularly long spell, she declared in an almost whispered voice, "This year I think I'm turning twenty-one." She died within the next two months.

BEGINNING ASSUMPTIONS

As we move through the experiences of our lives, many of us find, upon reflection, that we have some basic assumptions about what it means to be young, to be middle-aged, and to grow old. Many of these assumptions about aging were learned when we were very young. Some of our understandings have developed from experiences with immediate family members and other older persons. Others have become part of our way of thinking as a result of tales we have heard about older people. Many of these tales are filtered through newspapers, magazines, and television. Especially influential assumptions about aging and old age arise from the astounding absence of focus on healthy and active elderly persons as a whole.

This book is about aging and elderly people. It is filled with their stories and the experiences of working with and caring for them. It is also filled with suggestions for caregivers who are in the process of learning how to improve their efforts to help aging and dying elderly persons. By helping persons work more effectively and caringly with elderly persons in an agency, nursing home, or perhaps other health care situations, we provide for a better standard of living for all of us.

Since many professional caregivers are caring for their own family members, this book will be useful at a personal level as well as for helping others. Some caregivers who are reading this book may be entering middle age or approaching their middle sixties. These persons may find that they are thinking of themselves and where they are in their personal and private journeys. Others, such as young caregivers, may be confused and frightened by their experiences of working with elderly persons. They may find that grief education and working with elderly people will cause them to begin thinking about the aging and possible deaths of their family members. Every caregiver goes through stages and times when grief education and experiences make it difficult to examine personal mortality issues. This is understandable since grief, loss, and aging happen to all of us. In this light, I hope the material presented here will be helpful to individuals, family members, caregivers of all ages, and members of churches or other caring communities.

Everyone Has a Story

Another assumption of grief education is that the latter years, which are referred to as old age, are a unique period in an individual's life. Old age itself is a story: it is a specific time period that is especially unique because of its richness of tasks, challenges, and opportunities. That is why this book is filled with vignettes, composite case material, and poetic pieces; its purpose is to bring to life the stories of elderly persons and their caregivers.

One of my favorite images of old age and the process of aging is that of a rich tapestry. As a collector of antiques, I am well aware of how old tapestries are highly valued for the pictures they portray. The picture, or scene, comes through even when the tapestry itself is a little worn around the edges. Well-loved tapestries are cherished for their history, as well as their deep, rich, and muted color combinations. In a similar way, old age can also be a treasure.

The tapestries of old age are likely to be found in stories as well as in old, and sometimes faded, pictures. This is fortunate, for it is well known that elderly people generally like to tell stories. Usually these stories are quite egocentric: older people tell stories of conquests and misfortunes; conversations revolve around their physical trials and emotional struggles. In fact, there is a story for everything!

Instead of referring to these stories as ramblings, living in the past, or repetitions without change, I assume that every person's story is a shared treasure. Further, I have found it helpful to refer to each person's story as part of a tapestry. I first came across the image of tapestry in connection with aging processes while reading the work of Ebersole and Hess (1990), two writers in the field of gerontology. They compare aging to "an intricate tapestry—consisting of threads of feelings, thoughts, desires and actions!" This combination of thoughts, feelings, desires, and actions comes to the attention of caregivers in the form of story. The stories or life tapestry of most elderly persons include unique experiences of grief and loss, death and dying, bereavement, and aging.

This tapestry image of old age has a functional as well as an aesthetic use in caregiving and grief education. For example, by examining a large number of experiences, we can form even larger tapestries that represent old age. From these larger tapestries, we are then able to tease out a number of threads (thoughts, feelings, and responses) that are held in common. These threads can then be rewoven to form the foundations for even more focused conversations concerning aging and caregiving.

Grieving Is a Spiritual Story

A third assumption that this book makes about grief education is one that is woven into the grieving process itself. This assumption is that, at its core level, grieving is a spiritual process. The spiritual process of grieving is alluded to by the Psalmist (30:10-11) who refers to grieving as the "changing of clothes of mourning into garments of joy." For many persons, the combined processes of aging and grieving are woven into the wholeness of life by the faith in a merciful God who hears our needs and helps us transform our sadness and mourning into joyful emotion. In the midst of this faith-filled experience, the focus of caregiving, as it pertains to persons who are in the later stages of life, is the healing and transformation of each individual spirit.

The overall tapestry of eldercare is based on the mutual efforts of the helper and the individual who is helped. The spiritual core of grieving, as story, is transformed when these mutual efforts are lifted up and shared in moments of caring. This experience of mutuality is an incarnational, or human-divine, experience. By this I mean that both mutuality and spirituality are to be found in the experience of being human. It is God who joins the human experience and helps us through processes of mourning and aging. As a result of the combined efforts of caregiver, elderly person, and the Divine Spirit, we are able to face the challenges of life, and of death, with dignity and spirit.

THE ROLE OF PERSONAL EXPERIENCE

Because grief and aging are personal experiences as well as professional fields of study and practice, this book has its roots in my own personal and pastoral experiences of mourning and grief.

Therefore, some of my own story is woven into these pages as well. This is part of the risk and the value of becoming a grief educator and a pastor to elderly persons, their caregivers, and their families.

In 1986 I began working at New Hampshire Hospital, a state-owned psychiatric facility with services for children, adults, and elderly persons. I had recently left the associate pastorate position in a local church to become a chaplain. I was newly divorced and suffering great emotional pain from that separation. I knew enough about grief to know that I was thoroughly disorganized and confused, emotionally and spiritually.

A short time later, a number of professionals, including myself, identified the need for the development of supportive programs for staff who worked in the nursing home units. It was my task, as a member of the Department of Pastoral Services, to design and lead workshops on the themes of grief and loss as well as related areas of stress management, handling change, and promoting self-care for caregivers.

Somewhere along the way, I became aware that this task of teaching and learning about grief and loss was not only helping others but was also helping me. I found that I was slowly recovering my life and finding a new focus for my ministry. The new paths were sometimes painful, sometimes exciting, and often challenging. Somehow, I found strength to teach, listen, pray, sit, give good-bye kisses, and do memorial services.

During these years, my mother, birth father, and two favorite aunts died. Other losses occurred in my professional life. Many residents and patients died too; most, but not all, died from old, old age. Staff and colleagues also faced traumatic losses through accident, major illness, infant death, old age, and suicide. In the midst of all this, I gained a greater understanding of the nature of loss and recovery and learned about some interventions that frequently help and responses that tend to be less helpful. Patients, staff, friends, and relatives taught me about living, grieving, and dying. They have been essential partners in this learning process.

Grief work is always grounded in personal experience, for one cannot educate without being educated! As such, my story also is one in which I hold a mirror before myself, as I note many physical, emotional, and spiritual changes, for as I continue to work with people of all ages, I realize that I, too, am growing older. For example, my eyesight has shifted several times, and I now need reading glasses all of the time. I have developed a chronic disease, late-onset diabetes. (This particular disease is found, without exception, in all of the women and some of the men on my birth mother's side of the family.) I am reminded of these and other changes due to aging as I write the chapters on aging, loss, grief, and bereavement and especially when I lead workshops.

It is fundamentally true that life, with its successes and failures, losses and gains, becomes subject to a review process for each of us as we enter middle age. This process is important in middle age; it is essential to those who are growing old. Through the life review process, we learn about our attachments to people and things, our losses, and the challenges, successes, and changes we have experienced.

Knowing that grief is a natural and healing process often comforts grief educators, caregivers, and counselors. It is a comfort to know that this process is a gift from God. It is a comfort to know that, no matter how painful the loss is, one can experience healing and growth. In the process of teaching, learning, and experiencing grief, our spirit touches that of our loved ones and finds meaning in the all-embracing spirit of God.

THE ROLE OF GRIEF EDUCATION

Grief Education for Caregivers of the Elderly builds on experiences gained through the training of caregivers of an elderly population in a psychiatric nursing home facility that is part of New Hampshire Hospital in Concord, New Hampshire. Here, the staff found that working with ill, aging, and dying persons and their families was extremely rewarding, although very stressful. As caregivers, they often faced personal and professional losses, perhaps for the first time, while in this caregiving environment. The support provided through grief education was therefore essential for new and experienced caregivers alike. This training was most helpful when the caregiver was able to express personal feelings; talk about beliefs and experiences; learn about biological, psychosocial, and spiritual responses of grief and phases of bereavement; and apply these understandings and insights to typical caregiving situations.

CONCERNS ABOUT AGING

Concerns about growing old and being old are not new to our society. Literature throughout the ages provides glimpses into the problems and joys of aging. What is new about aging in this generation is the sheer growth in numbers of people who will live to grow very old. What was called old age two hundred years ago is now middle age. Today, "old age" is divided into the three categories of young-old, middle-old, and old-old, spanning from 65 to 100-plus years! At New Hampshire Hospital, over a five-year period, 69 percent of the deaths occurred among the elderly population on the long-term care unit. Most of these persons were between 75 and 103 years of age. Health care services for this population are not adequate to meet the growing needs of elderly persons, their families, or the community, nor do we have sufficient understanding of their emotional and spiritual issues. We have come a long way, but we still have a long way to go.

HISTORICAL TRENDS AND ELDERCARE

Three trends have an historical impact on work with the grieving elderly: the growing professional field of gerontology, the study of grief, death, and dying, and the emergence of trained mental health professionals. These developments have all had a profound effect on eldercare.

Historically, the study of the phenomenon of aging—gerontology—is linked with the National Social Security Act of 1935, which recognized and made provisions for the "elderly" in our society. At this time, age sixty-five was set as the age for retirement and Social Security benefits. This assistance was particularly important during the Great Depression when additional resources were scarce.

Concurrent with the rise of the field of gerontology has been the emergence of the growing field of grief study. Two research projects mark the beginnings of this field. The first event that helped establish grief as a recognized area of study was the Coconut Grove Nightclub fire in Boston. Follow-up research done by Eric Lindemann, in 1942 through 1944, described the grieving process of family and survivors of this tragic event. A second research project was conducted by Elisabeth Kübler-Ross, in the late 1960s in Chicago. This project also was a field study focusing on emotional responses of dying persons. This pioneering research still guides us today.

A third trend, particularly in the fields of sociology, psychology, nursing, and pastoral care, has been the recognition of the need for mental health professionals who are trained in gerontology and in working with dying and grieving persons. This training is very much in its early stages, as is evidenced by the experiences of caregivers who participated in the workshops that are the basis of this book. In this sense, the material provided here is part of the continuing endeavor to provide better care for elderly persons.

THE GRIEF EDUCATION WORKSHOP FORMAT

Purpose

The purpose of the grief education workshop format, as referred to in the following pages, is threefold. It provides an opportunity for clergy, colleagues, interns, and others to learn and grow in services and in ministry with the elderly. It is a vehicle for enhancing elder-care and for supporting highly stressed staff. Furthermore, this format provides the opportunity for dialogue with colleagues and students, toward the mutual goals of advancing learning and insights about grief and bereavement care for older persons.

Goals and Parameters

In the following pages you will find several workshop models for caregivers of the elderly. These focus on the themes of loss, grief, and bereavement care. The quality of care of elderly persons in health care facilities depends on the training and support of its caregivers. The contents of this book will provide the basic resources for training caregivers in the area of grief and loss in this type of health care community. This book uses the workshop and in-service model prevalent in most hospitals and nursing homes. The material should be adaptable to other settings, such as acute care hospitals, retirement communities, hospice and home health care, and churches. Although much of the didactic material (concerning bereavement and death and dying responses) shares a commonality with all stages of the life cycle, the major emphasis of this work is on processes and caring interventions for those in the young-old, middle-old, and old-old stages of life.

The Workshops

Each of the ten workshops opens with an exercise to orient the individual participant to his or her feelings about and experiences with loss, aging, and dying persons. These exercises include grief history surveys, attitude checklists, videotaped media representations of death and dying, and visualization exercises of self as an aging person. People are encouraged to share their beliefs and concerns with one another during this time.

The second component of each workshop is the provision of didactic material. This material is given in lecture format and typically includes one or more of the following: the normative development and issues of old age, the normative grief responses and stages that a dying person goes through when facing death, phases of bereavement, and caregiving goals and interventions. Each of these themes is based on the biological, psychosocial, and spiritual needs of the elderly person who may be dying or experiencing other losses.

A third component of each workshop design is the opportunity for caregivers to practice what they have learned in the workshop setting. Case studies, participant-generated problems (both personal and from the work site), simulated role-play, and the design of team care plans, as well as open discussion, are used to provide opportunities for caregivers to work with the feelings, experiences, and material presented. Each workshop ends with the completion of a workshop evaluation sheet.

Primary leadership for these workshops can be provided by personnel from one or several professional disciplines. In the models used, pastoral services personnel designed and led or co-led each workshop. Chaplains, nurses, parish clergy, social workers, and psychologists are encouraged to work together to provide a multi-disciplinary approach to grief education. The assessment and discussion of educational needs is presumed to precede the design of any workshop. This can be accomplished jointly with nursing and other departments. It is also important to have other persons involved to aid the registration process, help make referrals, and cosponsor the program. Workshops ideally have a minimum of two leaders, one male and one female.

Workshop Feedback

Each workshop begins with stated objectives and concludes with written evaluations by the participants. Leaders are also encouraged to evaluate each workshop at its conclusion, making note of changes that would be helpful in future endeavors. The feedback collected over the last twelve years has been the basis for the content, style, and leadership design presented here.

A second source of feedback is likely to come from increased calls for pastoral care regarding grief and loss experiences. Related to this is the increased use of chaplains and other clergy or pastoral care persons as consultants on treatment planning teams and in special incident reviews. The importance of these trends is not so much the increased use of chaplains or clergy but the growing recognition of the importance of a holistic approach to grief education and bereavement care.

A third type of feedback is to be found in the incorporation of an educational program, such as the one presented here, into the routine of the hospital, institution, or agency. When this happens, leadership teams can be identified and formed based on growing competencies. This constitutes the next step in program design and shows increased willingness, knowledge, confidence, and commitment to grief education. Paying attention to administrative feedback is a third essential layer to the provision of quality educational services.

Grief Education Assumptions

Education always rests on certain assumptions that may be explicit or implicit in nature. Nevertheless, grief education is best served when as many assumptions as possible are made explicit. The following assumptions, therefore, reflect an understanding of both the challenge of and mandate for grief education for all persons working with elderly people.

It is essential for a caregiver to understand that:

- *Life is a process of physiological, psychological, sociological and spiritual growth.* Old age is an identifiable, developmental stage of life. In this sense, growing old is more than degeneration of the body and preparation for death. Further, the old-age phase of living has characteristics that are common to other stages as well as those unique to old age. Unresolved issues and successes of previous stages become part of the aging process in the later years.
- *Bereavement and grief reactions are opportunities for psychological, sociological, and spiritual growth.* These processes and responses naturally move toward integration and recovery.
- *Caregivers can learn and grow in their caregiving capacity.* This growth can lead to better interventions and enhanced caregiving relationships.
- *Clergy have a unique and socially honored role as grief educators and caregivers.* Therefore, it is essential that clergy be trained for their role in caregiving for elderly people. Other caregiving professionals need to be trained about the inclusion of clergy at appropriate and helpful caregiving moments.

AN OVERVIEW OF THIS BOOK

The grief education resources presented here are designed to provide caregivers with a practical sample of what can be done and how to engage in grief education in their own settings. Each chapter builds on the contents of the preceding one. At the same time, one can begin anywhere and move from one chapter to another, as long as all components are eventually addressed in the educational program.

Beginning with Chapter 1, "The Challenge of Grief Education for Caregivers of the Institutionalized Elderly," grief education is viewed as a resource for enhancing the lives and functioning of elderly persons and their caregivers. This is particularly true when the effort combines the needs of the elderly with the commitment of the institution and the resources of caregivers. The goal of grief education, as defined in this chapter, is helping persons live lives that are meaningful to them and helping individuals meet loss and death in ways that provide personal integrity and relational wholeness.

The realities of old age are often clouded in mythology and misperception. The challenge of grief education is to provide a better description of the process of aging. Chapter 2, "Aging and the Elderly," describes some of the challenges and experiences of old age. Using Erik Erikson's psychosocial model of human development, old age is presented as a time of introspection, wherein the individual begins to review personal history and to have feelings about it. This introspection can lead either to despair or to integration.

In Chapter 3, "Bereavement and the Elderly," bereavement is described as the phases that individuals go through as they grieve the loss of a significant person in their lives. The works of Eric Lindemann, John Bowlby, and J. William Worden are the foundation for describing these phases, tasks, and grief reactions. Knowledge of the phases of bereavement is an essential component of grief education.

Because we live in a society that has been able to conquer many of the diseases and hazards of living, we have been able to significantly lengthen the individual life span. At the same time, death has become removed from much of our everyday living. Chapter 4, "Death and Dying and the Elderly," examines death and dying from a developmental point of view and focuses on emotional responses and phases of dying. Research pioneered by Elisabeth Kübler-Ross and Avery Weisman has been crucial in focusing research on the dying experience.

Chapter 5, "Workshop Design—A Successful Model," is meant to provide encouragement for others to engage in grief education. Material presented in this chapter is based on what has been learned from conducting actual workshops. Grief educators are instructed to consider issues of mission, goal setting, program design, and other components for running a successful workshop. A conceptual base or framework (such as that presented in the preceding chapters on aging, bereavement, and death and dying) is very important. The process of leading training programs is a learning experience for leaders as well as participants. Therefore, workshops that are truly successful will evolve and change over time. The training and approach of the grief educator is considered essential to running a successful training program. The complexity of the leadership role is stated as follows: *The leader of a grief education workshop is ideally a caregiver, a counselor, and an educator.* The complexity of this role is spelled out in this chapter and in the two subsequent chapters.

Caregivers (according to what we have learned from persons in the caregiving field) underestimate their presence in the caregiving event. Yet, the observer and the event are always interrelated. Each affects the other. This means that in grief and loss, as in all caregiving, the caregiver is essential to the caregiving event. The caregiver's use of self is an area that is yet to be fully developed as a dimension of care for the elderly.

In Chapter 6, "Caregivers: Practitioners, Helpers, and Companions," a model of care is presented based on the changing needs of the elderly person. This enables caregivers to feel empowered to move through a helping system that is based on resources and roles that have been thoughtfully reflected upon and carefully chosen. A section focusing on obstacles to caregiving identified by caregivers who work with elderly persons is also included. This chapter ends with some thoughtful questions that are intended to draw the caregiver into more personal reflection. Two essential areas for self-reflection are identified: motivation to be a caregiver and strategies for self-care while caring for other persons.

In Chapter 7, "Clergy As Caregivers," clergy are described as caregivers who are able to bring meaning to the lives of colleagues and elderly persons in sorrow. In this light, pastoral strengths, limitations, and other obstacles to caregiving are reviewed as helpful sources of personal assessment. Knowledge of oneself as a pastoral caregiver is essential for provision of pastoral care to elderly persons.

This chapter concludes with the suggestion that clergy see themselves as Recovered Healers. The image of the Wounded Healer, as coined by Henri Nouwen (1979), focuses on the grieving capacity of the clerical person. Yet, the goal of grief work is rightly seen as recovery, or fullness, of life. Therefore, a fundamental shift from woundedness to recovery is an important reclaiming of a valued concept. Recovered Healers are caregivers who have struggled with personal grief, who have recovered or are recovering, and who choose to journey with others who are also grieving and hoping to recover. These are people who, in ever-increasing self-awareness, are able to embody an ever-present faith amid the challenges of life and death.

Because work in this field is so urgently needed, the final chapter, "Envisioning Eldercare," examines the future of eldercare. This material is presented in an effort to offer points of dialogue. The complexity of issues in the field of caring for elderly persons cannot be too highly estimated. There is much to know and even more to discover. Feelings are often passionate when conversation turns to the question of resources for the growing number of aging individuals expected in coming years. Ethical issues are more and more commonly a routine part of daily discussions at home as well as in institutions and other care situations. How can we not consider eldercare an important issue for our day? Today we speak of eldercare as caring for others, but we know, deep inside us, that tomorrow eldercare is about caring for ourselves.

Chapter 1

The Challenge
of Grief Education for Caregivers
of the Institutionalized Elderly

I first started clinical work at New Hampshire Hospital in the summer of 1982. As I listened to patients and residents, I became aware of what it meant to them to be mentally ill and hospitalized. It seemed that much of their world was centered around an overwhelming experience of loss and grief. They would speak daily of loss of home, vocation, family and friends, church and faith, health and individuality, freedom, and hope. Frequently, I would hear about the time, precious time, of which their illness had robbed them. Often they spoke of the loss of their youth, of middle age, and even of seventy years spent in the hospital. This pervasive sense of loss and grief was confirmed by the experiences of students in our clinical pastoral education program at the hospital and by the experiences of others such as chaplains and staff. To be mentally ill is to experience not just the ordinary losses of living but the extraordinary loss of an all-consuming illness.

In August 1985, I joined the hospital staff as Protestant chaplain and then as director of the Department of Pastoral Services. Now, more deeply involved in direct pastoral care throughout the institution, I worked more frequently with the elderly unit. It was at this time, during the final moments of a patient's life and the days following, that I observed staff doing their best to provide quality care for these elderly persons.

Just as loss and grief were prevalent among patients of all ages, so too was their toll great among caregivers. Here, in the elderly unit, caregivers were faced with the stress of working with an aging and institutionalized population, with multiple health problems, and minimum or no social supports. Some patients slept much of the day. Others were fed through tubes. Others were lost to the realms of dementia or the final stages of Alzheimer's. These persons were not dying from the pains of mental illness but from age—from sixty-five to one hundred-plus years of living!

For example, it was during this time that a ninety-seven-year-old woman died. The last time I saw her alive was about seven o'clock one evening, when I stopped in to see how she was doing. I had never heard her speak. The week before, I had been at her bedside when her only son, approximately seventy years old, had come by to visit. The nurse on duty at that time appeared relieved to refer him to me, since the son was having great difficulty visiting his dying mother. At that time, he shared with me that he had not lived with his mother since he was a toddler. She had nearly scalded him while giving him a bath. She had been hospitalized, mostly in a psychiatric facility, since she was twenty-seven years old—some seventy years. She no longer knew him and had not for some time.

He had visited her infrequently over the years because he could not handle her craziness and rejection. Now it was his responsibility to make arrangements for her burial and to be with her while she was dying. He had selected a funeral home but confessed that he wasn't up to being alone with her. It was then that I offered to be with him and to work with him to provide a funeral for her.

Later, at her graveside, twelve formerly estranged relatives (from nine to eighty years of age) and two staff persons participated in her funeral. On a beautiful fall day, under a huge maple tree, we said good-bye. She was surrounded by family, most of whom had never known her, and two staff members who had represented her surrogate family for seventy years. Back at the hospital, the staff confided that they were angry that the family was there but had not come to visit her while she was alive. I, on the other hand, had celebrated that her son had come and that, before dying, she had looked up at me with big blue eyes from under a beautiful comforter that a caring staff person had drawn around her. I thought it was wonderful to see generations gathered round to hear what she was like in her life and to come together, even at this time. Some had not spoken to one another for years!

The countryside was remote and beautiful, and having grown up on a farm, I couldn't help but appreciate the beauty of the day, the site, and the persons. The family was appreciative and talked to one another. Meanwhile, the staff remained angry and bitter and distant. I knew that they were grieving. I also knew that their intense grief was affecting the care they were providing to this family. Their grief blocked them from being supportive of the family during this time of need. I wondered how many of these conflicted feelings would be carried back to the unit to affect their work with other residents and families. I knew something needed to be done.

GRIEF AND LOSS SUPPORT SERVICES NEEDED

In the fall of 1986, the staff of the Department of Pastoral Services met with the chief executive officer of the Psychiatric Nursing Homes Services to discuss ways to support staff in their grief over the death of patients. From that meeting came the proposal that Pastoral Services provide staff workshops on "death and dying" and "grief and loss."

The first workshop was held in the winter of 1987. It consisted of the sharing of personal experiences of loss, a presentation on normal and complicated bereavement responses, and a case example focusing on interventions related to grief and loss. Between 1987 and 1990, ten workshops were held, with 108 participants representing all caregiving fields within the elderly services unit. More workshops were held from 1990 to 1995. Today, grief education is an integrated part of the total health care program.

THE SCOPE OF THE NEED

What began as an identified need for support for caregivers working with elderly people who were facing death and/or grieving, soon began to take a specific shape. The identified need of "support" was found to have three components: administrative, educational, and therapeutic. These three areas provided the challenge and the parameters of our workshop focus.

Administrative Support

None of these workshops would have been possible without the explicit recognition and support of the chief executive of the unit. Through this channel, the area of need was legitimized as important and, more than that, as essential to meeting the needs of the patients. The challenge included the allotment of time, the legitimization of need, and the provision of services through the educational in-service model. We were fortunate that administration saw the need and presented the idea to us at a time when we in the department were similarly focused on grief education. From this and other experiences, we have identified that the basic requirement for administration is to have a clear concept of grief education and a means of naming and supporting training in this area. This is a fundamental challenge in all grief education efforts in institutions.

Educational Support

The second challenge, that of the provision of support through the in-service educational model, was actually the easiest of the three challenges to meet. The hospital already had a format for skill acquisition in place. Further, stress management and grief education were recognized as essential interventions, based on observed burn-out rates, high staff turnover, and management problems with individual patients. These tangible observations provided the motivation needed to develop a grief education program. Staff turnover and burn-out on the old-old age units were particularly high.

After the first workshop, our hypothesis was confirmed: staff, in general, did not have a working awareness of the grief process or of normal responses to death and dying. At this time, we were also aware that the staff needed to practice applying the fundamentals of grief process theory to specific case situations. The challenge of educating the staff about grief and loss processes and relating this to an elderly population was enormous.

Therapeutic Support

The third identified need was for therapeutic support. A portion of what was identified, by the administration and the Department of Pastoral Services, was the underlying goal of support through knowledge and acquisition of skills. An equally important dimension was encouraging caregivers to talk about what happened during their day, about patients who were critically ill and facing death, and about how they felt and how they, too, grieved. It seemed that if staff were supported, quality care would occur as a result. However, here, too, we faced a challenge not uncommon to caregivers and to grieving, that of avoiding focusing on oneself by keeping the focus and the feeling on the patient. An equal part of the challenge was the difficulty caregivers had in identifying either too closely or not at all with the aging and institutionalized person. We found that aging persons, their grief, and their death can be very threatening to their caregivers.

In summary, the challenge of grief education for caregivers of elderly persons consists of providing support through administrative, educational, and therapeutic foci. There must be time to talk about death and dying, grief and loss. Caregivers need to hear from one another, to affirm, support, and challenge one another in practical ways. Training should be available for caregivers in grief work, focusing on skill attainment, practice, and maintenance of skills. Caregivers must identify and enhance their role as supportive persons. Further, there is the need to identify and affirm the individuality, personality, and level of experience each person brings to the job and to the educational effort.

A MANDATE FOR GRIEF EDUCATION

The obligation to provide grief education for caregivers of the elderly comes from the needs of the elderly, who face the grief of aging and loss (including the anticipation of their own deaths). The mandate also stems from the obligation of a healthcare facility to provide the best care possible for the aging client. This means that the caregiver must receive the following training components:

- A working theory of aging, death and dying, and grief and loss
- General information about the needs of the grieving elderly person, with attention to specific living contexts (homes, assisted care, and long-term care facilities)
- A focus on appropriate caregiving interventions
- A means for support of elderly persons through an understanding of personal and professional responses to aging, dying, and grieving patients

Why Grief Education?

If the obligation to provide grief education arises from the expressed needs of persons working in the caregiving field, then the rationale for attempting to meet those needs comes from a broader understanding of the reasons for attempting this kind of education. The growing field of gerontology, the study of aging, the study of grief, death and dying, and bereavement, and the growth of trained mental health professionals were previously identified as major trends affecting the field of grief and loss education for caregivers of the elderly. More specific reasons for meeting the needs of caregivers and elderly persons and furthering the challenge and obligation for grief education arise from experience and observation in the field. Eight such reasons make grief education essential.

Knowledge about grief is helpful. The intellectual "knowing" of the universal stages and responses of grief tends to affirm and normalize the process of grieving, which leads, in many cases, to recovery with fewer complications. A review of research in grief and loss education indicates that the amount of education an individual has, in general, can be a factor in the potential for complicated grief (Glaser and Strauss, 1968).

Social changes tend to make death threatening to individuals. In our industrialized and medically advanced society, there exists a sense of continuous change. Viewed in this light, death can become one more experience of loneliness rather than a natural process, with continuity of connections and completion of social and individual growth.

The needs of seriously ill persons and the elderly in particular are great in today's society. Complex factors make it ever more challenging to meet the needs of seriously ill and elderly people. The sheer number of elderly persons and length of their life span is increasing at a faster pace than our knowledge of their health concerns and unique needs. We have relied on hospitals and nursing homes to provide for our elderly population and, in so doing, have lost some of our ability to value, care for, and live with these persons in our midst.

Early learning about death and loss often causes complications for the dying and the bereaved. Our first experiences concerning death and dying often come early in life and involve the media, pets, or our fears and fantasies of separation. If the death of a close family member occurs when we are young, this event is often considered something to hide from and may become a basis for further fears in later years. Grief education can help participants sort out these early losses and assist with grief recovery. This enables individuals to face grief in the here and now, with integrity of self and profession.

Education is a resource. As we grow and develop as individuals, we often learn from other people's experiences as well as our own. Much of this learning becomes a way of modeling that can be of great value. By providing structured experiences for learning, and by mixing beginning, intermediate, and advanced learners, the range of modeling opportunities expands greatly. This ability to observe and reflect upon what is modeled leads to professional and personal advancement. Therefore, persons in the field of grief education, in which growth and recovery are complementary goals, can use education as a professional and a self-help dimension.

Connectedness is essential to psychological, social, and spiritual health. It has been claimed that education is a great socializing factor, a bearer of social and spiritual standards in particular. Grief education provides the connections people need to recover from personal and professional losses for the sake of a greater standard—the ethic of helping one live and die with meaning.

Mental health and care giving professionals lack grief education training. Experience still indicates that most professionals are not adequately trained to work with dying and bereaved persons. Training in this area will empower these professionals to provide supportive interventions that improve the quality of life for the individual and increase self-esteem and reduce stress for the caregiver.

Grief education helps direct-care staff. In health care facilities, those who are often the closest to the dying or bereaved person are the nursing assistants. Yet, these persons may receive little help from other "professionals," who often are not confident in the field. Grief education, as demonstrated at New Hampshire Hospital, is one way to meet this need for training for all staff.

THE GOAL OF GRIEF EDUCATION

The goal of grief education is to help persons live lives that are meaningful to them and meet loss and death in ways that provide personal integrity and relational wholeness. Daniel Leviton has stated this goal in terms of enjoyment of life. "Death education, too, should have an ultimate goal—increased human happiness. Our goal is to help people understand their own feelings and attitudes toward death and dying so that death will be less fearful and living more enjoyable" (Leviton, 1971, p. 30).

Depending on one's philosophical or spiritual stance, the goal of grief education is to provide meaning, direction, and energy for life and for the completion of life with purpose and integrity of spirit. Objectives for such a training program must be congruent with the needs of the elderly, the functioning of the health care facility, and the training and support needed by the mental health practitioner or designated caregiver.

GRIEF EDUCATION OBJECTIVES

Although grief education necessitates covering some basic material, each training program is unique and must be treated accordingly. The training program developed in the Nursing Home Services of New Hampshire Hospital is an outgrowth of our specific needs, policies, and understandings of education and health care. Our process for development and support of staff includes the following general educational objectives:

- Provide quality patient care through continuing growth and education on the part of our staff.
- Utilize appropriate formal and informal educational opportunities as they arise in the training of administrative, professional, and support personnel.
- Set program goals that include:

  1. enhancing the staff's competency in meeting patient/resident needs,
  2. expanding staff knowledge and awareness of new clinical and administrative developments, and
  3. contributing to initiatives for optimal patient/resident care. (*New Hampshire Hospital Policy and Procedures Manual* [NHH Policy], 1997)

Grief education at New Hampshire Hospital has been provided in three formats: orientation programs for new employees, in-service training programs, and continuing education opportunities.

Orientation for New Employees

Orientation programs are means by which new employees are "provided with an overview of the hospital's mission, programs, policies and procedures" (NHH Policy, 1997). During the Pastoral Services orientation program, new employees are first introduced to the issues of loss and grief in a hospital situation.

In-Service Training

In-service training focuses on the "acquisition and/or improvement of competencies which are of immediate value to the service delivery capacity of personnel" (NHH Policy, 1997). During an in-service program of two to six hours, an employee receives instruction in the basic theories of aging, death and dying reactions, and grief and loss responses. This time is also used for employees to share their experiences and to discuss how these experiences, combined with knowledge of the grief process, can help them provide better care for the elderly.

Continuing Education

Continuing education consists of "education beyond initial professional preparation that is relevant to the type of patient care delivered in the hospital . . . provides current knowledge relevant to an individual's field of practice and may relate to findings from organizational improvement activities" (NHH Policy, 1997). In a sense, we make a distinction between in-service and continuing educational programs based on the length of time provided. When focusing specifically on continuing education, we often attempt to examine components of grief education in more depth, having assumed the basics of grief and aging theory. These topics include grief therapy, spiritual needs of the elderly person, expansion of caregiving interventions, and use of personal experiences of loss in the caregiving situation.

In summary, the challenge of grief education is to meet the individual needs of patient, caregiver, and institution in ways that better enable each person and facility to learn and grow from grief and dying experiences. The grief education goal for our facility can be stated as: the goal of grief and loss education is to provide optimal patient/resident care through enhancing staff skills and competence in meeting patient/resident needs.

Our organizational training objectives to meet the grief education goal are to:

- orient new employees to grief and loss issues for patients and residents within the hospital,
- use regular in-service programs to focus on the acquisition and improvement of the employee's ability to work with grief and loss issues as a service delivery component of the patient care plan, and
- provide regular continuing educational programs, focusing on increasing the effectiveness of the employee's capacity to meet the grief and loss needs of the patient or resident who is growing old and who may die while still a resident of the hospital facility.

Workshop objectives are to:

- grow in awareness and insight into issues of bereavement,
- develop a working theory of aging, grief, and loss,
- increase awareness of significant losses and anticipated losses in the caregiver's life, and
- sharpen caregiver intervention skills.

A diagram indicating the grief education training program's position and role in a hospital service delivery system for aging clients can be found in Figure 1.1. Here one can see the most important assumption of grief education for caregivers of the elderly in an institutional setting: a training program focusing on staff educational support regarding grief and loss can be directly related to the meeting of grief and loss needs of elderly patients.

FIGURE 1.1. Death and Dying, Grief and Loss Education

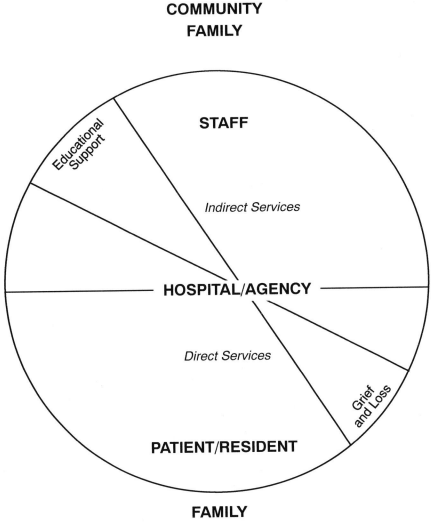

Chapter 2

Aging and the Elderly

Grief education, as an educational and supportive effort, must always begin with the needs of the participants in mind. In the case of training caregivers to care for elderly persons, the first essential focus must be on knowing the elderly person. The primary question is, "Who is the aging person and what are his or her normal needs?"

This is an ancient question. In the Psalms of the Old Testament, an aging person, as part of a life review process, calls upon God to address the continuity of personal need, amidst the aging process:

(An Old Person's Prayer)

In you, Yahweh, I take refuge;
never let me be put to shame.
In your justice, free me, deliver me!
Be a sheltering rock for me,
and a walled fortress to save me;
for you are my rock, my stronghold.
My God, save me from the hands of the wicked,
from the grasp of rogue and tyrant!
For you alone are my hope.
Yahweh, I have trusted you since my youth;
I have leaned on you since I was born.
You have been my strength from my mother's womb
and my constant hope.
I have seemed a mystery to many,
but you are my strong refuge.
My mouth is full of your praises,
filled with your splendor day by day.
Do not reject me now that my strength is failing.

> I am old, now my hair is gray.
> O God, do not forsake me;
> let me live to tell the next generation
> about your greatness and power.
> (Psalm 71:1-9,18)

The study of the phenomenon of aging, gerontology, has been growing by leaps and bounds, particularly during the past thirty years. As such, it has been part of other social efforts to provide better care for persons of all ages. One target population for better care has been the frail elderly. The sheer growth in numbers of this population and the stress that increase currently places on services for the elderly is expected to continue for some time.

As we consider the elderly in our midst, one of the problems we have to confront, as individuals and as a society, is our own bias about old persons. Many of us assume that people who are very old and frail are just "waiting around to die." This can be a common assumption of caregivers, family, and society. It affects, on multiple levels, what we perceive the aging person to be doing and/or what we think they should be doing. Common expressions of this agism (bias) are found in statements such as, "I wouldn't want to live like this." He or she "is just old and waiting to die." "Who would want to live to be ninety?" "If I'm that old, or that sick, just shoot me and put me out of my misery." These statements are often followed by more subtle expressions of avoidance, anger, and denial regarding the individuality and needs of aging persons.

The perspective of growth and recovery takes a different approach. It sees aging as a stage of life rather than a preparation for death. Although death is a certain and final aspect of the aging process, it is not the sole characteristic of it!

THE DEVELOPMENT OF LIFE SPAN PERSPECTIVE

By taking a chronological view of human aging, one sees birth (or perhaps conception) as the beginning of the developmental process and death as the end point. Between these two points are all the stages of life that we use as markers to discuss common psychological, social, biological, and spiritual developments. We may identify some of the following: birth, infancy, childhood, youth, young adult, middle age, and old age. The point is that life has a natural progression from one stage and time to another.

For the purposes of understanding the aging person, one must focus on that which makes the person distinct as well as that which he or she has in common with other age groups. The continuity of this process can be described within the parameters of birth and death. Today we are beginning to separate old age into the categories of young-old (sixty-five to seventy-five), middle-old (seventy-five to eighty-five) and old-old (eighty–five and older).

Characteristics of Life Span Perspective

There are three important characteristics of the life span perspective. The first is the belief that old age is best understood by viewing it as a phase or stage of universal human development. Second, it is understood that this phase has challenges and characteristics in common with previous stages and some that are unique to this stage. Third, it is assumed that issues which remain unresolved and successes which are accomplished at earlier stages factor into the success of the current, old-age phase.

CHARACTERISTICS OF OLD AGE

In 1959, Erik H. Erikson described eight stages of human psychosocial development. At that time, he also described eight crises that were characteristic of these different stages. In *The Life Cycle Completed* (1982), the eight stages and their related developmental tasks are:

- Infancy—basic trust versus basic mistrust
- Early childhood—autonomy versus shame and doubt
- Play Age—initiative versus guilt
- School Age—industry versus inferiority
- Adolescence—identity versus identity confusion
- Young Adulthood—intimacy versus isolation

- Adulthood—generativity versus stagnation
- Old Age—integrity versus despair

At the eighth stage of personality development, the individual must come to grips with valuing his or her life. During this time, nearing the end of life, the individual begins to review his or her personal history and to experience a variety of emotions concerning the past. Such an introspection leads either to despair or to integration.

When this process brings about integration the individual values his or her life positively, a result Erikson defines as ego integrity. When the individual recognizes the goals, failures, and ups and downs, as well as other events that make up the content of one's self, and affirms this as a whole life to be accepted, he or she experiences a measure of ego integrity. This is an affirmation of "I am me."

However, a similar life review can also result in doubt, fear, dread, and guilt. In this experience, the individual comes to a negative valuing of his or her personal life. The result is fragmentation, ambivalence, or ego despair. It is as though the person says, "I can not face who I am."

The challenges of old age, including changes, multiple losses, and in some cases, physical and mental deterioration, can stimulate a period of learning and growth, in which continued needs are met according to an appreciation of one's own selfhood. From a developmental perspective, the goal of life is the ability to cope with life and death with integrity, based on accepting one's self in one's own essence or spirit.

Butler (1975) described the developmental characteristics of old age as containing the following elements:

- A change in meaning
- A shift in perception
- An undertaking of a life review
- A desire to leave a legacy
- The establishment of a sense of serenity and a capacity for growth

DEFINITIONS OF AGING

The state of being old was defined by the National Social Security Act of 1935. In this model, age sixty-five was the entry point into retirement and therefore old age. When this age was set, there were fewer people living much beyond this point than there are today.

Old age is also defined by its end point—death! We have already dismissed this as an unhelpful definition, as we are beginning to see that there is much to do developmentally during a potential life span of some sixty-five to one hundred years.

A third way to define aging is to view it descriptively as a continuous and unique set of processes. In this descriptive focus, we can see that aging consists of biological, sociological, psychological, and spiritual processes. By knowing something about these processes, we can learn something about growing old and about the elderly.

THE GRIEF OF GROWING OLD

There can be no doubt that growing old has its rewards. From the perspective of old age, one can find meaning by looking back on personal, relational, communal, and spiritual experiences. These experiences can become sources of creativity and serenity in one's later years, and a legacy for generations to come. Each reward can be listed and treasured, as it should be for every life. However, growing old, in the middle-old and old-old years, is frequently experienced, even by the most buoyant, as a time of challenge.

A Disability Exercise

Imagine yourself as an old person. Let us say you are eighty-five years old. Imagine your ears being filled with wax so that you can hardly hear. Imagine trying to have a conversation over dinner with friends, when all you can hear is the sound of your own chewing as you eat a salad.

Imagine yourself sitting in a wheelchair, immobile from the chest down, wheeling with thumb and forefinger down a busy, narrow corridor. You are surrounded by others who are moving slowly and bumped by those who are moving more quickly.

Imagine yourself looking at a magazine, in a crowded doctor's office, and only being able to see the edges of pictures. Imagine the text looking like what you would see if staring through wax paper. This, and much more, is what an aging person may experience daily.

Among other things, old age can be experienced as an ever-building series of losses that may actually begin in middle age. "The griefs of growing old begin with the first realization that one cannot do, with ease, something that one previously had been able to accomplish without thought; that one will not, now, achieve the fullness of one's hopes and dreams; that one's life is not limitless, but finite, and that the time remaining is not great" (Raphael, 1983, p. 283).

The following poems describe two experiences of aging. The first focuses on an elderly patient with advanced dementia:

Randomness Is

No.
He cannot hear
or see
or tell
or feel the pain
when his arm is pricked.

And yet,
They say
just recently he used
to smile
and startle
and seemed to turn
when touched
lightly on the shoulder.

No more.
It seems
pictures of the mind
and
sounds of the heart
will never again meet
while his world
in randomness stands.

The second focuses on a man in his late sixties. He was not liked by many of his caregivers, who focused on some of the things he had done in his earlier lifetime. At this point, he had developed cancer and had a long history of alcoholism.

Here's to an Old Geezer

Well, there it is,
The time has come.
The heart can stand no more.
And so we sat
And talked a bit
Before we closed the door.

"I used to work with my hands,"
He said.
"I was proud of what
I did.
I've tried my best,
And I've made mistakes,
That's just the way it is.

Only now I'm ready and
It hurts a little.
But that really is okay.
Just sit right here
And be with me
For it's getting dark today."

The time has come.
The lamp is lit.
The hand in my hand
Is still.
Well, there it is.
And no more sound,
When we finally closed the door.

A DESCRIPTION OF THE AGING PROCESS

When we look at aging from psychological, biological, sociological, and spiritual viewpoints, we find this period marked by changes that we can use to identify with persons who are in the midst of this phase of life. First, we will look at the psychology of aging, as evidenced by the "aging brain" and by behavioral, perceptual, and emotional changes. Next, we will focus on the biological or physical aspects of aging. Evidences of sociological aging, including role and lifestyle changes, will follow the biological aspects of aging. Finally, a descriptive theory of aging must take into account spiritual changes and needs of the older person.

The Psychology of Aging: The Aging Brain

As a person ages, there are changes in intellect, perception, memory, and learning ability. Each of these changes can vary in degree. Individual management of these changes can be greatly enhanced by the appropriate pacing of tasks, provision of prompts, built-in motivational components, and the fostering of feelings of emotional security. As much as individual variation and coping can assist the aging brain, they do not change the fact that the brain does age.

For example, it has been noted that one in four persons over the age of eighty have dementia; of these, 50 to 80 percent have or will develop SDAT, or Alzheimer's type dementia (Tomlinson et al., 1970, in Levy and Post, 1982, p. 29). The impact of this is clear to younger persons, when we consider that one of four grandparents or parents may develop senility if they live into their eighties. Of course, conversely, this means that three out of four persons will not have senile dementia.

Cognitive brain changes related to the speed of mental processes also occur as a person ages. It has been shown that cognitive functions are 20 percent slower at age sixty than they were in the same individual at age twenty (Birren et al., 1979, in Levy and Post, 1982, p. 74).

Problem solving becomes a slower process with age. One apparent difficulty is the older person's motivation to solve problems, particularly those presented in testing situations. Another, very real perceptual problem is the aging person's decreased ability to weed out redundant information in a given problem (Mussen et al., 1979, p. 470).

Another important change in the brain's functioning for older persons is the increasing difficulty they experience with secondary or short- to middle-term memory (Mussen et al., 1979, pp. 471-472). It seems true that older persons can better remember what is happening in the present and what happened twenty to fifty years ago than they can what happened last year. Part of the difficulty of secondary memory relates to the issues of acquisition of new information and the retrieval of this information in a useful way. Knowing this, we begin to see how some of these changes in cognitive speed, problem solving, and memory can have an effect on the grieving process, which often presents itself as a difficult problem, with recovery taking a moderate amount of time.

Psychological Aging: Behavioral and Emotional Changes

The aging process presents changes in behavior, self-perception, and reactions to change in all the dimensions of an individual's life. People have feelings about what they can and cannot do, how their roles change, how they look and feel—aspects of their lives that are integral to their self-image. Physical changes often affect their life-style and their sense of attractiveness and prestige. One social confirmation of a person's age is retirement. Although people may look forward to this time, financial difficulties as well as a much-altered lifestyle frequently follow retirement.

Along with all these problems come issues of dependency and self-esteem. An individual may feel more dependent on others for daily tasks and relationships. This feeling of dependency may have associated fears and concerns about other changes to come. Elderly persons are brought up to value independence, work, and health, as well as aesthetics of beauty, sexuality, and self-determination. Psychological despair may result from feeling that some of these valued aspects of life no longer exist or need to be changed. Integrity can be found but only with psychological change. Coping and affirmation of self is always part of the task when biological and psychosocial changes occur.

Biological Aging

The beginnings of change (of emotional loss) are found in early middle age—perhaps with a change in weight, vision, hearing, joint flexibility, hair amount and/or color, and so on. It is an unusual person who does not at one time say, "I'm getting older." Even as we continue to grow, psychosocially and spiritually, we must admit that time changes our bodies, and that is not usually a change we take lightly.

A list of normal changes in an aging person's body can be extremely long and is itself a reason for examining the losses of age in relation to the grief response. Age brings thinning and/or loss of hair. The skin may become thinner, drier, and wrinkled and have age spots. Teeth may become infected and gums decayed, making dentures difficult to use. Movement may be slower and become difficult and limited. People actually lose height as posture changes. The voice may change, becoming huskier or very faint. Vision changes often occur in the early forties, and cataracts may develop as aging continues. It may become more difficult to hear the higher pitches of sound, and one may develop ringing in the ears or other hearing difficulties. Internal organs such as the lung, heart, and arteries may function in diminished ways. Hormonal changes may cause changes in sexual functioning. Muscles may lose some of their tone. All of this is usually a gradual process that may begin in middle age. Some of these changes are apparent in early old age, and many are present in the late seventies and eighties.

The most common physical problems of old age are illness and accidents. It is estimated that 80 percent of elderly persons have at least one chronic disease, such as diabetes, high blood pressure, arthritis, and heart and/or kidney problems (Mussen et al., 1979, p. 474). Old people are particularly concerned about colds, the flu, and falling and breaking a shoulder, leg, or hip. Many older persons are on medications and may have complications with drug interactions. Some have problems with ingested substances—alcohol in particular.

Sociological Aging

When speaking of sociological aging, one is describing role and lifestyle changes brought about through biological changes, social customs, and values. Social aging includes biases (agisms) that dictate that people should retire around sixty-five to seventy years of age, take time to pursue hobbies, get out of their children's hair, and be "good" grandparents. Those in big houses are expected to scale down, travel, and perhaps volunteer for charitable concerns. Today's society has included golf, quilting, gardening, reading, and sometimes a part-time job on a list of "to dos" for young-old persons. By middle-old age the individual is expected to appreciate the grandchildren or great-grandchildren, focus on the family, provide directives for his or her own death and the leaving of a legacy. These are generalizations, but they provide a realistic view of life-style and role changes that include family, communal, and social responsibilities and involvement and concerns about where one is, or is not, in society.

Spiritual Aging

Everyone has spiritual needs, which, as a person ages, become focused in five areas: philosophy of life, awe and insight into the numinous, relationship to a deity or higher power, relationship to nature and other people, and self-actualization (Beck, Rawlins, and Williams, 1988). As a person ages, he or she needs to identify, accept, and perhaps share insights in these areas because they, taken together, represent development of personal spirit and soul, an area in which individuals often find means and energy to integrate the other dimensions of life. Carl Jung (1933) called aging a process of individuation, wherein the person, particularly in the second half of life, begins to know his or her self (soul).

Spiritual aging includes facing issues of life, relationship, God, and goal achievements and failures. It also includes the all-important question of what happens at death, forcing one to examine personal beliefs about life, dying, and afterlife. One is also confronted with the loss of affiliations and access to activities. As the individual ages, those religious activities that once were available become out of reach to those who are ill, shut in, or frail. It is important for aging individuals to meet their spiritual needs. In some cases, these spiritual feelings and experiences are new for this phase of life and therefore constitute learning and growth.

EXPLANATORY THEORIES OF AGING

In considering the psychological, sociological, biological, and spiritual aging of human development, we have been presenting patterns that describe aging for many people. We believe these to be normative patterns of aging. The elements of growth and of loss are natural characteristics of the aging process. There remains the question of "why" people age. A list of explanations (see also Hess and Markson, 1980, pp. 18-21) includes the following:

Biological Answers

- Biological programming theory (aging genes)
- Wear-and-tear theory (the run-down clock)
- Decreased cell function (molecule damage and stress adaptation)

Psychosocial Answers

- Disengagement theory
- Activity theory
- Altruistic gene theory
- Reciprocity rule of exchange theory
- Symbolic interaction or personal meaning theory

Personality Answers

- Life span developmental theory
- Stability of personality theory

Spiritual Answers

- Wisdom and honor
- Afterlife and/or the kingdom within
- Self/spiritual growth and actualization

A look at the biological explanations of aging indicates that all three share the common assumption that aging consists of biological deterioration, making it difficult to know which is the most convincing argument. Even as we expand the length and often the quality of life, we cannot expect to live forever. All three of these theories remind us that we must deal with the physiological losses and grief of aging. Such losses and the resultant grief are particularly descriptive of this stage of life.

Psychosocial theories focus on meaning, relationship, and activity. Growth explanations, which are supported by this author, focus on aging as a process of development of reason and a means for providing the stability of social foundations, of sharing and relating in communal contexts. These theories suggest that this is what the individual is meant to be, to grow and develop and provide for the human community.

The most prevalent of psychosocial theories is the disengagement theory put forth by Cummings and Henry in 1961, which is still a popular theory today. It states that aging is a means whereby the individual detaches himself or herself from society. Presumably, this paves the way for new persons in new roles, within the species and the community.

Contrary to this is the assumption that aging persons still continue to be involved in activities throughout their life spans. What actually seems to be the case is that those elderly persons who experience meaning and value in their personal and social lives continue to be selectively engaged in that which remains or becomes meaningful to them (as long as they are physiologically and mentally able).

In discussing the aging personality, the author has already noted a bias toward the perspective of growth and individuation (selfhood) as the normative experience of aging, despite the challenges and physiological losses that come with advanced age. This theory is supported by Erikson (1959, 1982), Butler (1975), and Jung (1933).

What is rejected, however, is the second personality theory, which describes normal development as being fixed at a very early age, sometimes as early as three years old. This view, a legacy of Freudian theory, is probably a correlate to the biological explanation that views the aging process as a running down of the biological clock. Developmental perspectives and a descriptive analysis would indicate that the personality normally changes, grows, and develops throughout life.

Aging can also be explained within a spiritual framework. As people age, they develop insight into life and its meaning and direction. This insight can be valued (honored) by society, such as it was during the period covered by Hebrew Scripture. Here, society's value of the wisdom of elders was understood in the context of God's plan at work in their lives. This approach can be identified in other religions and cultures as well.

A second approach is found in the New Testament. It, too, sees aging as a spiritual process. As a person ages, he or she is expected to engage in spirit-filled relationships that progress toward a spiritual afterlife and/or a greater spirit of fellowship here in the "kingdom on earth." The early Christian church maintained the importance of living in the spirit, with Christ, and in the kingdom. All three are the goals of life for the mature Christian.

A third view focuses on spiritual growth through human development. This includes an emphasis on acceptance of self and the past as having value. Meaning comes from reflecting on life's accomplishments, relationships, and inner spirit. Aging persons do learn and grow. They do find meaning. Many do look to the spirit of the universe and/or the kingdom of God, and many also find the spirit of selfhood part of the process of aging.

In summary, as people grow old, they confront the challenges of old age, which include multiple losses and the ultimate task of reviewing their personal lives and finding meaning. At no other time will the urgency of these two tasks come together for such an extended and final period. To help aging people integrate these losses and challenges becomes the primary goal of caregivers.

Chapter 3

Bereavement and the Elderly

As a person grows older, challenges continue to develop, particularly in the areas of lifestyle changes, physiological changes, loss of friends and loved ones, and anticipation of personal death. Therefore, the second essential focus of grief and loss education is on bereavement responses of the elderly. A sixty-four-year-old colleague shared with me this feeling:

> It's not just that my parents are dead. They're already gone, along with my aunts and uncles, and all of that generation. Now my cousins are all gone too. I'm the next one to die.

Maintaining one's sense of identity and purpose is essential at all ages, but in addition to this, elderly persons often struggle with health issues and to maintain personal control of their environment. This aspect of aging may be particularly prominent in middle-old and old-old age.

UNIVERSAL BEREAVEMENT RESPONSES

The grieving response in elderly persons is similar, in most cases, to that of adult persons of any age. This response includes universal reactions, in typical phases, which are identified by specific mourning tasks. Most individuals move through these phases, complete the specific tasks of mourning, and pass through grief to recovery.

Definitions

Three terms are used, sometimes interchangeably, when describing reactions to a significant loss: bereavement, grief, and mourning.

- *Bereavement* refers to the overall reaction to the loss of a close relationship. It is a term used to describe patterns, phases, and/or stages that an individual goes through when grieving.
- *Grief* is the emotional responses or effects experienced while an individual is in bereavement. These responses include anger, shame, helplessness, sadness, guilt, and despair. Other responses are also found in a grief reaction, such as relief, peacefulness, calm, and release. The combination of all these emotional responses, during the time of loss, is the grief response or grief reaction.
- *Mourning* refers to the psychological, sociological, and spiritual phases one goes through when detaching from a relationship. In this sense, mourning can be used interchangeably with bereavement. Mourning has traditionally been used to describe social and spiritual rituals.

Mourning, bereavement, and sometimes grief (in terms of an overall response pattern) are used interchangeably in many cases. During these grief education workshops, for example, caregivers responded favorably to the universal term of grief and were less comfortable with the term bereavement. In addition, they persisted on using the term mourning to relate to social or religious rituals. Elderly persons, on the other hand, were more likely to use mourning to express phases, grief reactions, and rituals.

GENERAL OBSERVATIONS

Four general characteristics of the phases of mourning can be identified: mourning is universal, unique, time limited, and process oriented. These four characteristics are basic to all grief work.

Mourning and Loss Are Universal

All people experience loss, regardless of age. Many teenagers, for example, have faced a number of significant losses by the time they become teens. As we become adults, we experience more losses. Some are temporary, and some are permanent. These losses vary in degree of impact on our lives. Even though we know about loss, each new one catches us unaware. Thus, shock signals the beginning of a grief response. Each and every significant loss envelops the bereaved in a cocoon of numbness and isolation. Each significant loss leaves us feeling as though we are going through something by ourselves. Sometimes we feel as though no one else has had a similar experience—so great is the pain! Grief is universal, however: No one is singled out for tragedy.

Mourning and Loss Are Unique

Although it is reassuring to know that all persons experience grief and loss, this knowledge always remains in conflict with an individual's experience of his or her own loss and grief as unique. Humans do not grieve exactly the same way. Neither is one loss exactly like another. There are aspects to each relationship, and within each individual, that make his or her story personal.

Mourning and Loss Are Time Limited

Many people are afraid they will grieve forever, like a stream that runs into a neverending sea of emotions. Grief, however, is time limited; it is part of a universal timeliness. Just as "There is a time to every season" (Ecclesiastes 3:1), so too is there a certain amount of time for grief.

Mourning and Loss Are Process Oriented

Mourning is a process that has a beginning, middle, and end. For example, recently, a young woman in her early twenties called to ask for an appointment. A number of months earlier, she had experienced the loss of a client whom she cared about and for whom she continued to grieve. She had not been able to talk about this at the time of her loss but now came to say that she cried a lot and was depressed. She felt that she was not getting over the loss as quickly as her colleagues were. She talked and cried and remembered the relationship. She was able to say good-bye and to move on with her life. She claimed that it was most helpful for her to know that it was okay to grieve, that there are phases of mourning, and that it was okay to stop grieving.

WHY DO WE GRIEVE?

It is now possible to describe a normative grieving process for people of all ages. We are beginning to develop new theories about why people grieve. To understand why human beings grieve, we must understand something of the nature of loss itself. The question posed is, "What is loss?"

John Bowlby (1980) has provided an explanation for grief reactions, based on his observations of young children. According to Bowlby's attachment theory, all persons form attachments to their primary care-takers, usually a parent. We are not alone in this bonding; other species do likewise. This closeness of relationship provides emotional security and meets practical safety and survival needs. Any threat or loss to this parent-child relationship causes panic, anxiety, sorrow, and anger. When loss occurs, a distinct grief reaction is observed that includes four phases: numbing, the urge to recover the lost person or object, disorganization and despair, and reorganization. The separated child's first goal is to recover the relationship. Grief reactions are a working through of this separation.

GRIEF AS NORMAL LIFE CRISIS

On a larger scale of human experience, grief can be seen as a normal life crisis. According to developmental theory, there are normal crises in life that are typically manifested at specific stages of personality development. Grief, as a life crisis, is found in all stages of human development. Old age is a period marked by a great number of significant losses. At the same time, to be emotion-ally connected with significant others remains a natural and essen-tial part of life; it is the purpose and role of these connections that change as we mature in age. Physical changes, illness, and stress, combined with significant loss of personal relationships, are fairly common crises for aging persons.

BEREAVEMENT STUDY

The earliest systematic study of grief is attributed to Eric Linde-mann (1944) and his study of fire victims in a Boston nightclub in

1942. He interviewed survivors and their families and loved ones. Lindemann was interested in the phenomenology of grief. He wanted to know what happens to people when they experience the loss of a loved one through death. What do they think? How do they feel? How do they behave? What happens over time? Grief, as a result of Lindemann's research, can be described as normal responses to death caused by painful separation from significant persons in one's life. As a result of this study, grief was described according to symptoms and emotional responses that occur in fairly typical sequences during a critical period of time.

TYPES OF LOSS

Lindemann's work was focused on acute and traumatic loss. Since then we have learned more about other kinds of loss. Some of these losses were mentioned in Chapter 2. The most significant losses associated with aging were described as physiological loss and losses pertaining to role, relationship, and community. As a person ages, these losses tend to be abundant and often permanent. It is the abundance of loss and consequent lifestyle changes that complicates old age.

THE TASKS OF MOURNING

J. William Worden (1982, pp. 11-16) described four tasks of mourning:

- Accept the reality of the loss.
- Experience the pain of grief.
- Adjust to an environment in which the deceased is missing.
- Withdraw emotional energy and reinvest it in another relationship.

General grieving processes typically follow this sequence. Experiencing the pain of grief, however, appears to be part of each of the other three tasks. The pain comes and goes, in waves of greater and lesser intensity. However, each of these tasks, though difficult, can be accomplished by most individuals. Elderly persons, while continuing with the usual grieving process, may also have modified responses that can be considered normative for their age group.

Task 1: Accepting the Reality of the Loss

Society structures its rituals to reinforce the personal acceptance of the loss of a loved one. The processes of disposing of the body, informing friends and relatives, placing the obituary in the paper, and holding the funeral or memorial service all help the bereaved person know that the deceased no longer physically exists. These social tasks and observances are recognized more quickly than are intrapsychic and spiritual processes.

Accepting the reality of the loss means acknowledging that reunion is impossible. The bereaved tests this reality through searching behavior, which often leads to misidentifications and calling out for the deceased. Resistance to accepting the loss is a natural part of the grief process: denial, avoidance, and attempts to bring the person back through extraordinary means actually leads to acceptance of the reality of the loss in most cases.

Task 2: Experiencing the Pain of Grief

Early in the grieving process, limits are placed on the expression, intensity, and nature of personal grief. Customs, regulations, and church and family systems that are usually valued by the bereaved can be influential in setting these limits. Sometimes these norms may inhibit the bereaved in meeting personal needs. The bereaved individual may feel unable to express personal pain when faced with comments such as "Men don't cry," or "It's for the best," or "One must move on in life." Further obstacles to experiencing the need to grieve may involve expectations about a spiritual afterlife and that one should be joyful, the custom of returning to work quickly, and the practice of not talking about painful subjects a month or two later. Recovery from grief always involves accepting the reality of loss and the experience of pain from that loss. Experiencing the pain of loss, as stated previously, occurs in varying waves of intensity.

Task 3: Emotionally Breaking the Tie with the Loved One

Accepting the reality of the loss is a time-consuming process because the bereaved must fully withdraw his or her emotional energy from the relationship. In the case of long-standing and intimate relationships, it may take months for realization of loss to occur and for necessary adjustments to be completed. Spouses often find that at least a year is needed for adjustments to changes, such as moving, sleeping alone, preparing taxes, or vacationing alone. Anniversary dates and significant life events may continue to reactivate grief for some time.

Elderly persons also need time to adjust to an environment in which a spouse, intimate friend, or adult child is missing. Sometimes they choose not to internalize the loss and continue to experience that loved one as remaining near. Many look forward to reunion in an afterlife. It is common for dying and aged persons to be ready to die because they know they will be with their parent or spouse. This choice can be common among the middle-old and old-old population, so common that it may be normative of their age group. Elderly persons both accept the reality of the loss and, paradoxically, keep the emotional tie to their loved one in some spiritual way.

Task 4: Reinvesting Energy in Other Relationships

Most people move emotionally from loss, through grief, to recovery and reinvestment of energy in other relationships. At this point, the deceased person and that relationship become part of personal experience and memory. In recovery, these memories influence the person in a holistic sense rather than being a center of focus.

The following poem describes the process of forming new relationships and finding new meaning in life. This aging husband visited his wife several times a week for the sixteen years that she was hospitalized in a psychiatric facility. He has moved on with his life and no longer comes to the nursing home.

The Lover

He visits her as weeks go by
And feeds her oh so gently.
Years have passed

And he's used to it,
He says to me,
Matter-of-factly!

I see him often,
Lending a hand,
And talking to the others.
While he's been here
He's made more friends
Just by being kinder!

Her eyes are blue,
The color of sky,
Her hair brushed snowy white.
A sight she is,
Of luminescent beauty,
A star amidst the night.

No one more beautiful,
I must confess,
Is on this ward today.
Both he and she
Have made it so
For that is just their way.

It seems that in
Some other life
They laughed and loved
A lot,
And held each other,
In the good times,
As well as in the not.

But now she's gone,
With her strand of pearls,
And he comes to visit others.
No wife to feed,
Or sit next to,
His love moves ever outwards.

The withdrawal from memories of and desire for the deceased person is essential to recovering from grief. Most people experience anxiety in facing a world without the deceased. Feelings of guilt may cause this process to go more slowly.

GRIEF WORK: HOW LONG?

During a recent staff meeting, a middle-aged woman became angry and frustrated, declaring:

> All this talk about death is depressing. I've had all kinds of therapy and it didn't help. I'm still going through the same stuff anyway. I think only time does any good.

She was right and wrong. We cannot predict with certainty the length of time it will take an individual person to complete the tasks of mourning. Neither can we accept the belief that "time cures everything." Grieving and time use independent measurements. Time cannot be the sole measurement for grieving. Time is neutral. Grief, however, does take time. A significant loss may take from one to several years to be resolved. Reactions to special events and anniversary dates may still be common beyond that.

FACTORS THAT AFFECT THE COURSE OF GRIEF

There are a number of factors that affect the outcome of the grieving process (see also Sanders, 1989, pp. 15-17). There are four factors that I find to be key indicators of grief recovery for elderly persons:

- Nature of the relationship
- Nature of the loss
- Physical, psychological, sociological and spiritual condition of the survivor
- Resources available to the bereaved

The Nature of the Relationship

In considering the relationship of the deceased and the bereaved, it is helpful to consider the following:

1. The *number of years* the relationship has existed affects the grief process. Losses in old age tend to be associated with long-standing relationships that have emotional, social, and symbolic importance to the bereaved.

2. The *degree of function or dysfunction* of the relationship is an important factor in the course of grief. Elderly persons who watch their spouses gradually age and decline in health and activity may be more likely to be prepared for the death of the loved one and to see it as a blessing. In very dependent relationships, the bereaved may feel too threatened to continue on in life. In relationships that have been plagued by abuse, there may be some ambivalence, anger, and guilt about the relationship. This may be a family secret that has been kept for a very long time. Elderly persons often are afraid that other family members or outsiders will discover their "dirty laundry" during the mourning period. An older person will have great difficulty, for example, if the community members gathered at the wake or memorial service discover that:

   George was an alcoholic who drank up all the family money and beat Mary. He did this for years.

3. Losses of *siblings and adult children* are also factors when another significant loss occurs. Whenever there are losses which cause the bereaved to be the last living person in the family or which invert the natural age order of living and dying, the course of mourning is affected. It is devastating to outlive one's children, no matter the age! It is equally devastating to be the last of a nuclear family. As one alert ninety-six-year-old woman put it, "There were twelve of us children; now I'm the only one left."

4. Another consideration is the *degree of differentiation of roles.* Elderly people who can work through their grief by accepting the uniqueness of the deceased in the relationship may tend to have a less complicated grief outcome. Elderly persons tend to have time-honored family roles. At its simplest and most profound level, the issues of driving, cooking, repairs, peacemaking, intimacy, and finances all affect the course of grieving.

The more rigid the roles, the more likely the grief process will be difficult.

5. Considerations of *communication and unfinished business* are key indicators of the grief outcome. Planning and preparation for aging, dying, and after-death arrangements, as well as communication about beliefs, can help facilitate the course of grief. Elderly persons worry when "things" are not planned, and "not taken care of," so most elderly people discuss their wants and needs ahead of time.

The Nature of the Loss

Other factors determining the outcome of the grieving process have to do with the timing of the loss, the type of loss, and the number of losses the bereaved has experienced:

1. The *timing of the loss* can be particularly traumatic during certain life cycle transitions. For example, the beginning of retirement, the birth of great-grandchildren, and on or near the fiftieth anniversary all are particularly difficult times for loss to occur.

2. The *type of loss* is also an outcome factor. As can be expected, chronic and painful illness, accidents, and sudden death are difficult to handle. Elderly persons are afraid of pain, long painful illnesses, loss of self-control and decision making, and deaths they consider to be stigmatic from a social or religious viewpoint (such as suicide or attempted suicide). If the bereaved can perceive the loss as natural and timely, then his or her recovery is likely to be more normative in outcome. When death is prolonged, sudden, unusual, or socially less acceptable, then the process becomes more complicated.

3. The *number of losses* that the elderly person has experienced may affect the course of grief. Multiple losses, occurring close together in time, in one's personal life history and across generations, tend to create a sense of being plagued by tragedy.

The Condition of the Survivor

The degree of inner and outer correspondence of grieving and bereavement is a factor in the outcome of the grief process. This correspondence or lack of it is felt on biological, psychological, sociological, and spiritual levels.

1. At the *biological level,* the course of grief is affected by the perceived and/or real health of the bereaved. The fact that the bereaved is the same age or has a similar illness as the deceased will be a factor in how he or she identifies with the deceased. The degree to which the bereaved is able to manage daily needs is also important to outcome, as is the use or misuse of drugs, food, or alcohol.
2. *Psychological factors* include the person's emotional capacity to do grief work. Those in poor mental health, with low self-esteem and ego differentiation, may find themselves more depressed by the loss. Those who are ambivalent, angry, and guilt-ridden may have difficulty grieving. Elderly persons often experience feelings of anxiety, loneliness, and vulnerability. These feelings are often translated in terms of safety and security issues.
3. *Sociological considerations* have internal dimensions also. Elderly persons may have fixed self-images that are dependent on role and relational experiences with the deceased. Family rules and rituals can affect the course of grief in a positive way, when they meet internal and social expectations of the bereaved and his or her family and community.
4. *Spiritual factors* that can affect the course of grief are belief in God, a positive view of afterlife, and the ability to find meaning in a life without the deceased. Those who have specific ways in which they are supported may be uplifted spiritually in their movement to recovery.

The Resources Available to the Bereaved

Resources can be people, objects, beliefs, and tangible networks for meeting daily living needs in a timely and reasonable manner. The degree of change and availability in a number of resources will affect the degree to which the loss is experienced as a global life deprivation. Elderly persons who experience isolation, major lifestyle changes, and a poverty of communal and intimate relationships will find the course of grieving difficult. The basic needs of safety, security, and self-validation (meaning and identity) are all essential to good recovery.

PHASES OF BEREAVEMENT

Bereavement can be viewed as a series of phases, each one following the other in a somewhat predictable pattern. Four such phases can be universally discerned in ordinary grief reactions (see Bowlby, 1980, p. 85):

- Shock and numbness
- Disorganization
- Reorganization
- Recovery

Phase 1: Shock and Numbness

The shock phase begins when one learns of the death of a significant person in one's life. The individual experiences the blow or impact of that information on all levels. People often say the news hit them like a ton of bricks and that they couldn't move. The first response to a loss is a sense of unreality, of being frozen in time. The individual is now in bereavement. He or she may experience cognitive confusion, restlessness, feelings of helplessness, free-floating anxiety, and general emotional flux. Psychologically, he or she draws inward to an egocentric position. Spiritually, there is a sense of awe over that which is uncontrollable—the forces of life and death, the will of God, and creation.

This startle or alarm response may be followed by somatic symptoms, such as dryness of mouth and throat, sighing, loss of muscular power, weeping, trembling, sleep disturbance, loss of appetite, nausea, pain in chest or throat, difficulty breathing, and general aches and pains. These reactions are natural and protective, a way of managing a seemingly unmanageable situation.

From the beginning, family and caregivers help by providing practical assistance. The bereaved benefits from being helped to make decisions and provision of basic care needs.

For several weeks, bereaved persons may go about the tasks of living as though they were in some shadow of the real world. There is often a mechanical, robotlike, feeling about everyday events. Specific tasks to be performed vary, depending upon the degree and type of predeath planning.

Spiritually, the bereaved may turn quickly to recitations about beliefs, memorized prayers, and faith in the "afterlife." The first moments, even days, of numbness may be broken with a spiritual protest—"Why?" This may be addressed to God directly. It may be easier at this stage to "fuss" with God than with doctors, nurses, family, and self. People seem to know instinctively that life, death, and meaning are all in question. Other glimpses of feelings may surface, briefly, particularly in cases of unexpected or unwanted death. Most of these feelings are held in check by the numbing process. People say of their numbness, "I'm just going through the motions," "I can't feel anything." "I'm numb all over." This period may last from one to several weeks. Again, practical assistance is usually offered and most helpful at this time.

Phase 2: Disorganization

The awareness of loss begins gradually. After the funeral, the bereaved may have a wide variety of responses. He or she may experience separation anxiety and not want to be left alone. He or she may cling to other loved ones. With awareness may come intense feelings of anger, guilt, frustration, shame, and fear of death and life, of God and the Fates.

The bereaved may feel open, unprotected, and oversensitive to the environment in which the loved one is missing. There is searching, scanning, and pining activity, as the environment is actively explored in search of the loved one. Hopes of reunion are prevalent. Many of these responses are denial and disbelief, and they are normal.

During the beginning of this phase, the bereaved may do what is expected of him or her. This may be a mitigating response, while the actual grief work of searching and longing for the loved one continues. Numbness may come and go. Time remains somewhat suspended.

The search for the departed may also include a search for reasons for the loss. This existential "why" may continue, and even grow, as awareness of the magnitude of the loss heightens. This phase may last for weeks and even a few months. Listening and gentle affirmations are usually helpful during these early days of loss.

This second phase is a stage of disorganization, often referred to as "crazy time." Everything feels mixed up. Problems are likely to be exacerbated by issues of everyday living. One woman in her fifties described her experience:

> The day after the funeral, I got a call from my mother's landlord, telling me I had to get things out of the apartment immediately. The last five months have been just crazy. My house is filled with all her things. I even bought her a card for Mother's Day and she isn't even here.

Additional stresses are banks, bills, charge cards, and probated wills.

Emotionally, it just hurts! Feelings that the bereaved never knew he or she had begin to surface. Physically, the bereaved may go from no energy to excessive energy. This stage can be quite scary for the bereaved and difficult for caregivers and relatives/friends who have their own grief, although they may be less affected by the loss and therefore recover more easily.

During this phase, elderly people are particularly likely to place importance on transitional objects. This is not unique to this age group but may be an important factor to consider. Pictures of the deceased tend to be put away for a while, particularly current pictures, while those of earlier times may still be displayed. More likely an object, such at the deceased's pair of gloves, may rest nearby or even be worn for awhile.

Elderly people also tend to "behave by habit" during this time. This may continue for an extended period, as the relationship is often one of long standing. The table may continue to be set for two, the bed may be turned down for the deceased, or his or her clothes laid out. Family may be told to do things because the deceased would have done or wanted it that way.

A common characteristic of this stage is the need to tell and retell the story of the loss. Every second is likely to be reviewed again and again. An example of this is found in Chekhov's *The Cabman*, who tells each fare that his son has died (Chekhov, 1986). Elderly people appear to do this for a greater period of time than other age groups.

Some of this may be related to long-term memory prevalence, difficulty with problem solving, and sorting names, dates, facts, or feelings under pressure. That connection remains to be investigated.

The early part of this phase is marked by cycles of numbness mixed with wide varieties of feelings. The middle part is evidenced by equally mixed-up behaviors, including searching for the deceased and avoidance of reminders and tasks. Later on, a time of withdrawal and depression sets in, signaling internal grief work in which the bereaved begins to review the relationship. This may include talking through events and feelings. It may also be a very private experience, depending on the bereaved individual's personality. Toward the end of this phase of life and faith review, there usually is an unconscious decision to remain in grief, to regress in fantasy, or to change, grow, and live. Most people choose the latter and very gingerly move toward reorganization, the next phase of mourning. It is important not to underestimate the time needed for life review and decision making. The choice to move on must be an internal choice. Helpful interventions continue to be listening, encouraging expression of grief, and support. Many bereaved persons need protection from the extreme decisions they are likely to make during this time.

Phase 3: Reorganization

During the process of reorganization, the bereaved moves toward a world in which memories of the deceased are cherished in the absence of the physical presence of the loved one. This is an enormous task. During the early period of reorganization, waves of despair, lack of direction, and disorganization are mixed with occasional peacefulness and less intensity of feelings connected with the deceased.

During this time, a new reality must be affirmed. This reality may include new interests, new friends, and new roles. These changes may feel as if a wholly new identity is being formed. This is a tenuous time for the bereaved, who may find the restructuring of his or her inner and outer world too painful and therefore avoid the task. For example, I recently had a call from a widow of eight months who claimed that she was still not able to look at all the cards and letters she had received following her husband's death. It seemed to her that others were sending their pain to her, and she said she could not bear to have them do that. I suggested she hide her letters in a box for the present. They were still in hiding one year later. Her depression was just settling in as she faced the unconscious choice to stay in grief or to reorganize her life.

In summary, grieving has a turning point at which a decision is made to relinquish old roles, assume control over personal and social identity, and restructure and reaffirm the faith that new life is possible. However, this can take several years. Usually the restructuring of identity increases energy, levels of functioning, and hope. It is important to encourage, listen, and talk about the past, present, and future with the bereaved. Gentle confrontation may be helpful so that new possibilities and new resources can be found.

Phase 4: Recovery

It is important to declare a "recovery" or an end to grief. Even though the ending is not as clear as the beginning of grief, it is of great personal and clinical importance. People want to know that there is an end. They also want to know what that end might look like for them.

From the beginning, the grief process has been moving toward a goal of psychosocial, spiritual, and physical balance. Recovery is, therefore, a subjective response and a personal affirmation. For elderly persons, it generally resembles the ego integrity described by Eric Erikson for old-age personality development. When one has recovered from grief, one is able to live with the vicissitudes of life, to learn, grow, and affirm one's self. This comes from a life review process that includes experiences on all levels. Recovery embraces a complexity of tensions often described as "me as I was, am, and am willing to be."

What causes a person to let go of the role of bereaved? There is no single answer. The ability to relinquish this role may come from the everyday tasks of life such as learning a new job, earning the household income, mending the door, or painting the walls without assistance. Sometimes it is sitting in the church pew alone and asking oneself what one truly believes and having an answer or faith in a forthcoming answer. Often it is being the only grand- or great-grandparent or downsizing one's needs and home that aids this transition.

Recovery includes a new awareness of self, the assumption of responsibilities and acceptance of life without the deceased. Recovery frequently means acknowledging that the one who is beside me now is "spiritually" beside me, in the lives of my grand- and great-grandchildren or in the scrapbook of my mind. What is helpful at this stage is everyday relationships of give-and-take. The normalcy of life itself, including reciprocal relationships, helps the bereaved to heal.

EFFECTS OF BEREAVEMENT
ON ELDERLY PERSONS

Murrell and Himmelfarb (1989, pp. 171-172) studied the "Effects of Attachment Bereavement and Pre-Event Conditions on Subsequent Depressive Symptoms in Older Adults." This study has important implications for those who tend to see the elderly as too frail. What Murrell and Himmelfarb found was that older adults are quite resilient to the stresses of life changes. This means that bereavement effects are short-lived, usually largely dissipated within a year of the death of a significant person. Not surprisingly, however, older adults with weaker resources are more vulnerable to multiple life changes within a short period of time.

A second general observation about grief responses of elderly persons is cited in Raphael (1983, p. 311) who mentions the increased use of health care resources by bereaved persons during the fifth to eighth months of bereavement. This may indicate that elderly persons may be more likely to use health concerns as a way of addressing grief issues.

General Observations About Widowhood
and the Elderly

We can be optimistic about the generally positive recovery most individuals can expect after a significant loss. At the same time, it must be said that widowhood represents a prevalent and difficult situation for aging persons. Apart from the loss of an adult child, or the facing of one's own mortality, widowhood can be the most difficult situation faced during a person's later years.

Widowhood is linked frequently, but not exclusively, with aging and the elderly, and it is most appropriate to consider it a woman's issue at this stage of life. Widowhood is most frequent among women, who tend to have a longer life span than men and who are slightly greater in number in the general population.

Widowhood or widowerhood often represents an accumulation of losses, such as health changes, financial pressures, questions regarding living arrangements, changes in other relationships, and social isolation resulting from no longer being part of a couple. Often, the aging couple or individual may anticipate the death of a spouse and make plans ahead of time. Still, this accumulation of losses is a factor in successful grief recovery and a general characteristic of the elderly age group.

The first year following the death of a spouse is stressful. The bereaved may face financial problems, a new home, and living alone, sometimes for the first time in up to fifty-six-plus years. As a result of grief, loneliness, and anxiety, the individual's health may suffer, and the bereaved elderly person may die at an earlier age. It is typical for an elderly person to be functionally bereft without his or her spouse and to describe this loss in terms of how to carry on in everyday life. It is more normative for this age group to not express excessive yearning for the spouse's return. What is more often expressed are questions such as "What will become of me? How will I do this without him or her?" It is because of these practical needs and feelings that the aging widow or widower may move soon after the spouse's death to be nearer children or to retirement communities for assisted living and security.

Common symptoms during the first month of bereavement are crying, depression, sleep disturbance, decreased interest in life, lack of appetite, tiredness, and loss of interest in television, news, friends, and clubs. The leisure activity of just sitting and thinking, or general contemplation, common among the middle- and old-old age groups may now change to fitfulness.

The elderly may worry about what they did and did not do. They may have felt hampered in relating to the deceased by their own limitations and/or illness. One-fifth of the bereaved elderly have some degree of guilt over what they could have done (Cummings, 1969, in Mussen et al., 1979, p. 464). Some continue to directly or indirectly express this perception to others for a long period of time. As one sixty-eight-year-old woman exclaimed, "If only I could have seen, but I am blind. What could I do?" Her husband had fallen next to their bed and died immediately.

Despite all of life's complications, the months go by, and there is a gradual reorganization of life. The following are common characteristics of grieving elderly persons:

- They commonly see a doctor for help.
- They are the most apt to receive medication for grief reactions.
- They are the least likely of any age group to receive the proper amount and type of help needed.

According to Weiner, this is a major scandal in health care today (Weiner et al., 1975, in Raphael, 1983, pp. 311-314).

The elderly are most likely to hold on to the presence of a loved one (Moss and Moss, 1979, in Raphael, 1983, pp. 312-313), and they may do this for the rest of their lives. This experience is generally normal for this age group. However, individual monitoring and assessment is still essential when this occurs. Recovery for the aged may also mean holding on to memories, waiting for reunion in the afterlife, and maintaining egocentric positions regarding health and lifestyle.

Elderly persons, in general, are most likely to be conservative and to respond to learned social and religious conventions, even when they might privately consider or be encouraged to do otherwise (Mussen et al., 1979, p. 464). Remarriage during recovery can be quite successful for the elderly person, even though it is not often sanctioned by family and society (Mussen et al., 1979, p. 466). It is, however, not a realistic option for most elderly women because of their greater life expectancies.

Bereavement Complications

Most elderly persons successfully pass through bereavement and get on with their lives. Complications arise when an individual becomes stuck in any of the four phases and, after an extended time, does not move through to recovery. One complication, as mentioned earlier, is lack of perceived or actual resources. Elderly persons often have the least resources available to help them meet their needs in appropriate ways. As such, some individuals choose not to move on because the process is just too overwhelming without the needed support system.

We must remain sensitive to the choices made by elderly persons who wish to remain attached to a deceased spouse during their later years. However, we must be aware of dysfunctional grief, which can be generally defined as: "the intensification of grief to the level where the person is overwhelmed, resorts to maladaptive behavior, or remains interminably in the state of grief without progression of the mourning process toward completion" (Horowitz et al., 1980, p. 1157).

Complications with elderly persons tend to increase for men and for psychiatric and depressed persons. The first and last groups may suffer a fatal outcome from these complications, while the psychiatric population may experience prolonged grief. Older widowers tend to have increased morbidity during the first six months of grief (Raphael, 1983, p. 314). Elderly depressed persons tend to be higher suicide and attempted suicide risks (Shulman, 1978), and those with psychiatric problems may experience extended guilt (Parkes, 1983).

In summary, grief is a universal response to the loss of a significant person in one's life. It has typical phases and involves specific tasks. Most individuals accomplish these tasks and recover from their grief reactions. To do so, they must work through social, physical, psychological, and spiritual reactions and come to a sense of who they have been, are, and can be. This process is best described as a total life review involving an affirmation, and perhaps restructuring, of identity. Elderly persons may opt to hold on to images of self and the deceased, to a previous lifestyle, and to conventional values, even in the face of pressure to do otherwise. The demands of widowhood have been cited as an example of a typical loss for the aging person. Other losses include biological change, loss of friends and relatives, and occasionally the extremely painful loss of an adult child. Complications may arise in older men during the first six months, for elderly persons with inadequate resources, and for those who may have excessive and prolonged guilt, evidenced by abnormal self-reproach.

Grief is a response felt at all levels of human experience. Its manifestations are numerous. The spiral image found in Figure 3.1 demonstrates the movement of grief response from the most private to the most public expressions and feelings. For recovery to occur, these manifestations of bereavement must achieve some balance and integration.

FIGURE 3.1. Manifestations of Bereavement (Levels)

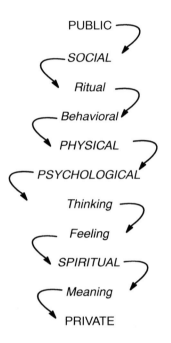

Chapter 4

Death and Dying and the Elderly

A third essential focus of grief education for caregivers of the elderly must be on the grief concerning contemplation of personal death. In no other age group is this issue a normative characteristic. Its role in the lives of the elderly is fraught with complex social, spiritual, and personal expectations. We who care for the elderly persons in our midst will never know for sure what this is like, until we are also aged and facing death. For this reason, it is imperative that we understand the process of grieving one's own imminent death in its normative pattern.

DEATH AND SOCIETY

Dying can be considered a personal, social, and cultural event. Often, what is experienced on a personal level is mirrored by social, cultural, and religious teachings. Every society has ways of teaching its members about dying and death. Some of our foci are the disposal of the body, disposal of the estate, support for the bereaved, and role allocation for family, job, and community, if necessary.

Death, we say, is the end of life, and we use medical criteria such as cessation of breathing, heartbeat, and pulse, as well as the onset of rigor mortis, marking the beginning of decomposition, and necrosis to identify it. Other criteria may be used to describe death. One such criterion is the departure of the soul from the physical body. Another criterion may be the degree of psychosocial and body function control. Clinical, social, psychological, anthropological, civil, and spiritual definitions of death have their own discipline-specific criteria.

DYING AND THE INDIVIDUAL

People who are in their older years die mainly because of physiological complications. For example, they may get pneumonia, and this, added to their other medical problems, leads to death. They may have a sudden heart attack and die. Elderly widowers are vulnerable to suicide, perhaps as a complication of grief. Others die from accidents and from a lack of will to live. We must not forget that there are different causes of death in old age, as in other stages of life. However, most old people die due to one or more chronic diseases or from multiple complications.

DEATH AND DYING: A DEVELOPMENTAL VIEWPOINT

Using the developmental viewpoint, aging and dying are described as part of a natural process. During old age, this process can involve diminishing physiological functions. Old age also brings increased integration, or selfhood, and a sense of meaningful life in relation to spirit and community.

Human needs are present throughout life, but the manner in which needs are met changes with age and personality development. Maslow (1954) described the universality of human needs throughout the life span. His hierarchy of needs is as follows:

- Biological Needs
- Safety and Security
- Belonging
- Self-Esteem
- Self-Actualization

These basic human needs are present in life and in dying. How well dying persons, family, and caregivers are able to meet these needs will determine the quality and character of an individual's dying and death.

DEATH AND DYING RESPONSES

Elisabeth Kübler-Ross (1969) thoroughly researched and described how persons respond to terminal illness. She was able to generalize these responses and to formulate the following descriptive theory of normal response stages for adults facing personal death:

- Denial
- Anger
- Bargaining
- Depression
- Acceptance

To this list, Parkes (1972) has added disbelief, jealousy, sorrow, and loneliness. Other responses can include apathy, apprehension, anticipation, and relief. The point is that each person has emotional responses to dying. Some are fairly universal, and others are unique to the individual's situation and personality.

In general, the five stages Kübler-Ross identified are helpful in understanding the differing individual responses to dying. Kübler-Ross understood that people follow their own timetable, that personality and situational factors may cause more of one emotional response and less of another. She defined five feeling responses to impending death:

- *Denial*—the "No, not me" initial response, includes shock and numbness and can be an important buffer time for a person who has just learned about his or her own impending death.
- *Anger*—the "Why me?" (frequently expressed to God) response, comes with the awakening of feelings, fears, and so on. Unconscious and conscious fears and fantasies are now fully functioning on all levels. This anger can include envy.
- *Bargaining*—the "Yes, me, but . . . " response, is expressed in the many subtle and direct ways the dying person tries to gain more time. These efforts may also be directed to God and the powers that be.
- *Depression*—the "Yes, me . . ." response, is often accompanied by a narrowing of focus and an emotional withdrawal, as the reality of death sets in intrapsychically.
- *Acceptance*—the final feeling response, is devoid of the intense energy and turmoil of feelings of the preceding stages. Energy is now focused on letting go and saying good-bye. (Kübler-Ross, 1969)

DYING WITH INTEGRITY

Each person dies his or her own death in his or her own way. We as caregivers need to know what that way is for each person. Sometimes, however, it is not possible to know fully what a dying person would wish to have done or not done. In situations such as this, there is advice to be found in research conducted by Hospice. This organization has published a Dying Person's Bill of Rights (Abbott, 1988, p. 15), which lists the needs and wishes of dying persons:

- To be treated as a living person
- To maintain hope
- To have questions answered honestly and not to be deceived
- To participate in decisions
- To express feelings
- To have choices
- To be free from pain
- To have loved ones receive help
- To share spiritual concerns
- To be cared for well
- To not die alone
- To be helped to live as normally as possible until death

Dying with integrity has been described as an appropriate death or a "good-enough" death, a term coined by Weisman (1972). It provides the following rule of thumb: a "good-enough" death is that which meets the needs of the dying person and which keeps suffering to a minimum.

Most people appear to have an inner timetable that may or may not afford a variety of choices and endings. Medical technology and dying in hospitals have brought added complexity to individual living and dying wishes. It can sometimes be difficult to accept choices made by the dying person. Nevertheless, some will choose how to die, as did this elderly woman dying of cancer.

No Heroics

No heroics
was what she wanted
and still the pain was great.
It was hard to say
who hurt the most,
she
or they in wait.

Patience, it seemed,
entered in
the hero of the hour.
Much in demand
to sit and hold
those gathered
round about.

No words
were crossed,
although
mumbles
grew,
as folks came
to say good-bye.

And the windows wide
were round about
as fresh air came inside.
No heroics,
just a gentle breeze
and sips
to ease the dryness.

Some will choose
to fight and spin,
wheels and tubes
and sounds
of metal things
to stir up life
impatient to be gone.

Yet
there she lies
with loved ones
round.
No heroics,
was what
she wanted.

Dying persons do plan their last months and hours, and make arrangements to meet their needs and their personal agenda. Some need help to express their desires and to work with family and caregiver agendas. One elderly woman discussed the manner of her burial and the nature of her memorial service. She spoke of these things to the chaplain within two weeks of her death.

Flowers on the Hill

Sometimes there is time
to sit and think
about what we want to happen,
of words to say,
and last requests,
and treasured memories,
passing.

Me, on foot,
and she, in chair,
we wandered
through the halls.
We talked of life,
we knew of faith,
and we planned the service all.

"Let there be mountains"
she said,
"and flowers on the hill,
and better yet,
don't forget,
those hymns
I love so well."

Then one day,
I was called,
to say a last good-bye.
We sat, I sang,
as hours passed,
songs
to light our way.

She was so gentle,
to the end,
I barely knew she died.
But then it dawned,
that she had gone,
to rest
upon the hillside.

THE DYING PROCESS

The emotional grieving process of a dying person consists of coping responses to three phases of dying:

- Beginning Phase
- Illness Phase
- Final Phase

Each of these phases is lengthened or shortened according to the physiological condition of the patient, the patient's attempts to alter the phase (will to live), and outside interventions (usually medical).

During the beginning phase, the dying person faces the threat of death. The person may know, or suspect, that she or he may be dying. Sometimes this knowledge builds over a long period of time. Still, internal recognition of impending death always comes as a personal shock, even for those with chronic illnesses.

During the illness phase, the individual's pattern of living may be altered due to physical decline. Frequently, these changes in lifestyle are frustrating. It may be difficult to ask for and receive help. There is increased anxiety and fear about pain, further complications, the presence or absence of a spiritual future and/or a legacy, and a concern for loved ones. Hope is mixed with despair. Denial, bargaining, and unresolved business make this a very difficult period, particularly if these reactions and responsibilities have not yet been faced.

The final phase occurs when death is expected within days. This phase is the most feared phase for dying persons, and it is associated with the most discomfort, although it usually is a time of the least physiological discomfort. This phase often leads to unconsciousness, followed by cardiorespiratory failure, as the heart stops beating and the lungs stop exchanging air.

TASKS OF THE DYING PERSON

Each individual must prioritize his or her own tasks when facing death. Some people will appear to have much to do, and some will have only one or two things on their list. Generally speaking, the dying person will include some of the following tasks in his or her goal of a meaningful or satisfactory death. The major tasks of the dying person are to:

- face impending death,
- maintain hope,
- manage discomfort and decision making concerning personal death,
- communicate needs to loved ones and caregivers,
- relate to loved ones,
- finish unfinished business and say good-bye,
- manage closure through affirmation of personal life meaning, and
- face an uncertain future with hope and faith.

COMPLICATIONS

Complications can add much stress to the dying process. For the elderly, complications are likely to be factors of time, resources, and treatment. It is very difficult to face a gradual decline in health that is mixed with relapses and changing hopes. Many elderly persons fear a slow and prolonged death most. Resources are also a problem for the elderly: medical bills, expenses in general, and wear and tear on the family through a lengthy illness and dying process are of great concern to elderly persons. Finally, treatment choices and hospitalization in an age of advanced technology make decisions difficult to control.

Some treatment choices have changed because of new technology. Certain surgical procedures are now more commonly available to persons in their advanced years. Yet, when an individual agrees to advance directives for care, he or she may be making decisions based on current knowledge, without realizing how rapidly medical technology changes from year to year. For example, one man died of a heart problem for which a procedure was available two years later. Other complications may involve cases in which technology is present and indicators for use are not strictly within the dying person's prerogative. Recently, the New Hampshire Hospital task force on end-of-life issues sought clarification concerning the question of a DNR order for elderly patients on community trips. It was discovered that paramedics are required to initiate CPR procedures when a 911 call has been made.

DEATH AND DYING AND ELDERLY PERSONS

Elderly persons face death in ways similar to other adult age groups. There are of course some differences. The older person, for example, is more likely to talk about death and to do so more openly and frequently. Death may also be addressed indirectly through questions about changes in the world, discussion of health problems, and comparisons with others perceived to be in similar, better, or worse health.

Aging people are apt to pay closer attention to peers facing death. They benefit from this modeling approach and use it as a learning experience. The extroverted elderly person, who is used to, and requires, feedback from others for self-understanding, can suffer greatly when models are ego-dystonic (too dissimilar) or are lacking. In this sense, elderly people benefit best from being around people who are their own age. Some awareness of this need is shown in the development of retirement communities, which offer continuity of care as the individual ages. The age-normative tasks of the elderly are assisted by a built-in mentoring process.

Of course, it remains true that facing death is more and more the task of elderly persons. It is not the sole task, but it is the final task of the aging individual. As fewer and fewer people die from illness, more and more will die from old age. Aging persons have to work through this final crisis.

Finally, the elderly are not necessarily ready to face death. It is not universally true that they are more prepared than any other age group. They have the same types of responses to death as other adults do. They may be ready, having done their grief work and made their preparations. They may be resigned to death and in some cases be depressed about it. They may avoid death, denying it right to the end. They have just as many types of responses to death as young and middle-aged persons do.

In sum, we need to pay attention to the elderly because they face death more frequently than any other age group, because of their specific needs, and because we know so little about them.

Dying and the Elderly: General Observations

Elderly persons are more likely to associate death with mental and or physical illness. This may be quite realistic because more old people usually die from age-related biological decrements than from a particular disease. These complications of aging are more likely to affect and produce problems with coping, reality orientation, and anxiety.

Elderly persons usually have a desire to leave a legacy, to resolve unfinished business and care for survivors. They may be concerned about themselves, that is, their physical pain and fears, but they want closure on relationships, and they want their lives to have meaning. The elderly person tends to focus on a mixture of practical and existential concerns when preparing for death.

Elderly persons need someone to listen to their hopes and regrets and to hear formal and informal confessions about their lives. The dying elderly individual's greatest fears are of abandonment, pain, and confusion.

Some have suggested that the older person has a natural tendency to consider himself or herself as younger than peers. This can be either a hopeful or a complicating factor in aging. It probably adds to denial during the early phases of decline, and it may lead to hope and energy as illness and the uncertain future draw near. Feeling younger than peers as a protective way to observe self and others, is perhaps a paradox because once again, the aging person is best helped by someone his or her own age. Intergenerational persons are less important to coming to grips with personal death.

To be beneficial, religion must be accompanied by the certainty of salvation. This is very important to the dying elderly person. As a sixty-three-year-old woman, a nonpracticing Unitarian, told me upon facing breast cancer surgery, "I do believe in God, Reverend!" In eight years, she had asked for prayers for others fairly infrequently, and this was the first time she asserted a certain belief. This came in the midst of what she felt was life-and-death crisis. A bargaining moment and an affirmed belief are the beginnings and the endings of grief.

Some elderly people seldom express serious concern about their own deaths. This appears to be true for the majority of elderly who are able to complete the phases, and therefore the tasks, of mourning their own dying. Others express great concern. There are a variety of factors that affect the dying person's grief process:

Age. It makes a difference whether individuals are young-old, middle-old, or old-old both in chronological terms and in the way the persons feel. Also of significance is how old their parents and siblings were when they died.

Sex. Males and females may not wish to live under certain conditions, notably the death of a beloved spouse. They may be suicidal. Men in particular are often depressed and will express a desire to stop living if they have survived a spouse in middle-old and old-old age.

Cause of Death. Few individuals want to have long, protracted, and painful life. When specific illnesses come, which are likely to be extended and lead to eventual death, many individuals will say that they are ready "to go." Elderly people are particularly afraid of dementia, including Alzheimer's disease, and painful cancer.

Ethnicity. Certain cultural groups have specific standards for old age and for dying; even the most confused individuals seem to have an internal clock that matches these norms.

Place of Dying. The issue of dying at home or in a hospital seems to be a concern for loved ones nearby; another concern is being kept alive as a "vegetable." People are afraid of the medical and legal professions and their desire to keep persons alive, even when they are old and ready to die.

Personality. A person who meets life's challenges and finds meaning in old age and in the summation of his or her life will be able to find meaning and dignity in dying. Those who lack meaning and resources will find the process more challenging.

Spiritual Beliefs. People meet the challenges of dying just as they have met the stages of living. Some aspects will be more challenging than others. Most people need something to hold on to in the way of meaning, relationship, and legacy. Most have questions of faith and afterlife. Working or not working through these questions as to the end of life and its meaning is a factor in the dying person's grief process.

DEATH AND THE LIFE CYCLE

How one faces death in old age depends on the degree of ego integrity (self-affirmation) or despair (self-doubt and judgment) the individual has at the time when dying is likely to occur. For those with ego integrity, death can be a blessing, something to face and talk about, to make plans for, and to accept. For those in despair, death can be feared. Death may be feared also by those who are not educated about it, by those who live alone, by those who feel rejected, and by those who have less belief in an afterlife.

In summary, older people have a more realistic perspective about dying than other age groups. This may be learned by paying attention to peers. It may also be a summation of the integrative life review task of old age. Nevertheless, the elderly go through personal grief responses and complete specific tasks so that they will be ready and able to face the very uncertain future, the personal end of life as it is known to them. Their biggest fear is of dying alone.

There are many ways to face life and dying. I have found that each individual has a certain dignity at the very end. Two closing poems reflect that perception. The first is about an Alzheimer's patient in her seventies who was a respected nurse in her younger years. The second was written after a sick call with a dying elderly gentleman.

She Used to Be

She used to be
a nurse down the way.
Family remember well
her last instructions.

Don't let me go there
to that place.
I'd rather die.
But come she did.
There was no choice
And no need to whisper,
Alzheimer's.

She would have said
the word

boldly,
clinician that she was.

In the end,
there was much to say
by those who loved her
and thought she believed.

But, who could tell.
She slept so much,
and snored so loud,
and made no trouble
anywhere.

Right to the end
she used to be a nurse,
and family remembered well
her last instructions.

A Call to Come

A call to come
Now or maybe tomorrow
life will change
moving
on to something new.
How to leave,
how to go?

No more strikes,
no blows to give, to those who
come too close, and ask too much.
Arms resting close,
fingers slower, barely moving,
lids that lift
to prayers and words
learned by heart, when
beating came more easily,

and time and space were more at one.
How to leave,
how to go?

A call to come
Now or maybe tomorrow
life will change
moving on to something new.
How to leave,
how to go?

Sounds of spoons
and squishy stuff
amidst a bed far down the way.
Quiet seems too large
a price
for some to go
and some to stay.

The task of dying appears to be a challenging one, with natural processes to lift the spirit and provide meaning to the event and to the life preceding it. Each person has an amazing ability to find this spirit and meaning. Those who have found meaning in the developmental challenges of aging will find meaning and dignity in dying.

Chapter 5

Workshop Design—A Successful Model

There is no one answer to designing a grief education workshop. Much depends on the purpose, goals, and expected participants. At the same time, it is possible to point to a number of essential components and to suggest ways these components can come together to provide a solid educational format.

In this chapter, the New Hampshire Hospital grief education model will be used to demonstrate what is involved in designing a workshop. This model and its variations have been successful at New Hampshire Hospital because they meet our needs. It is not, however, the only model. You, the reader, will want to develop the right program for your situation. You will want to consider physical and administrative atmosphere, your elderly population, and the particular needs of your caregivers.

The goal of grief education is to provide optimal patient/resident care through enhancing staff skills and competence in meeting patient/resident needs. To accomplish this goal, the following are appropriate participant objectives:

- Grow in awareness and insight into issues of bereavement.
- Develop a working theory of aging, grief, and loss.
- Increase awareness of significant losses and anticipated losses in the caregiver's life.
- Sharpen caregiver intervention skills.

Figure 6.1 in the next chapter demonstrates how these four components interrelate. This figure shows that the objectives cover the four learning outcomes of growth in theoretical conceptualization, insight, practice, and application of learnings in the caregiving context. All four of these learning components are brought together in the workshop—to provide a mini–life experience that can be used to review the past and provide for future life experiences.

WORKSHOP EXPECTATIONS

Each individual in a workshop brings personal expectations of what he or she believes is needed to make things better, given his or her specific situation. What is learned is often based on this anticipation of "pearls of wisdom." At the same time, educators may see these pearls as few and hard to come by. Nevertheless, the expectation of learning the extraordinary appears to be inherent in the workshop format. The paradox is that the material we provide is never that simple or that extraordinary.

What then can a participant expect to find? What can a leader provide in a workshop on grief education for caregivers of the elderly? One approach is to determine what the workshop will not be. It is essential to establish these parameters and to let participants know what they are from the start.

The workshop is not a case review, nor a clinical treatment team, nor a place for assessment, diagnosis, or the designing of an individual treatment plan. There is not enough time, structure, or information for a care plan. Nor is the workshop intended to be diagnostic, although there is the expectation that what is learned during the workshop can be used in diagnosing and devising individual care plans at a later time.

The workshop is not crisis management, nor is it a "cookbook" for how to provide counseling. Hopefully, participants will get some concrete ideas for interventions that will be of practical use in their specific situations. Still, the issue of "how-to" in a "recipe" format is not possible because there is never a single answer or only one way to be a caregiver.

The workshop is not a quick fix. This means that one, two, or six hours will not provide all the input needed to train caregivers. It takes time to become trained in the field. To know about grief and loss and about elderly persons, one must be continually involved in the learning process, as described in Figure 6.1.

The workshop is not therapy. Although participants do experience support and often resolve personal grieving issues during the educational process, the workshop is not structured for grief counseling. Those in need of such counseling may be referred, gently, as appropriate.

A SUCCESSFUL PROGRAM

When one approaches grief education for caregivers of the elderly, there are five factors necessary for a successful program: theme, participants, location, leadership, and format.

Theme

In this model, the general theme grief and loss education for caregivers of the institutionalized elderly was determined by expressed needs of caregivers, by hospital administration, and by the Pastoral Care Department. The functional theme is staff support toward quality care for elderly patients facing aging, loss, grief, and dying. The three components of the theme have been addressed in the preceding chapters of this book: "Aging and the Elderly," "Bereavement and the Elderly," and "Death and Dying and the Elderly."

Thematic considerations of grief and loss are also grounded in the unique caregiving situation. Variations on the general theme of grief education are based on considerations of work and loss experiences, personality, and availability of resources.

Participants

There is a tendency for people who work with elderly persons to become frustrated with their work. Increased stress from frustration often causes caregivers to engage in agist activities (such as blaming, avoiding, and depersonalizing). This is not surprising considering the neediness of elderly persons and the personal and professional issues of caregivers. For these reasons, considerations regarding members and types of participants in a grief education program are essential.

In the New Hampshire Hospital model, registration was limited to fifteen. Our best sessions have been when registration has numbered from five to nine persons. It is a good idea not to have a workshop for less than five persons. The goal here is to provide a richness of support and input so that the caregiver can work with personal and professional issues. By using the range of from five to fifteen participants, everyone has the opportunity to talk and to listen. In addition, the leader can also be available as a resource and for referral purposes. This material is highly emotionally charged, and the leader has the responsibility at all times to be alert to the group emotional climate and to individual needs. Many participants who come (by choice and by referral) experience fear, anger, and other feelings, some for the first time.

A mixed-group approach works fairly well in most situations. When using this approach, it is important to include caregivers from all disciplines and in all roles. These heterogeneous groupings provide modeling opportunities. Those who are in other stages of grieving and have other experiences can help those who experience an intense return of their grief. Those who tend to avoid expression of feeling can also learn from those who are more expressive.

Location

Ideally, the program should be in a quiet place that is comfortable and conducive to movement and interaction. There should be ample space to place newsprint on the walls (to increase visibility of common information and for the gathering of ideas) and to have equipment such as projectors and chalkboards. In addition, the location should be an enclosed space so nonparticipants cannot disturb the group.

An environment conveying a sense of confidentiality is paramount, and it is wise to stress this confidentiality at the beginning of the workshop. Participants need permission to express themselves to learn and grow. Personal experiences of grief and loss do have a profound effect on caregivers and the work they do. Participants are therefore encouraged to engage the material presented in the workshop at personal and professional levels as they learn how grief affects the whole person.

Participants are referred to the workshop because of personal losses, the general demands of their professions, and specific professional issues. One participant described her involvement with both personal and professional insight:

> I just lost my father a month ago. I know that I'm not up to par with my work. But I'm just barely getting through the day. My supervisor suggested I come to this workshop.

In addition to confidentiality (privacy), and practicality of the location chosen for the workshop, the time allotted for the program should be uninterrupted. By having the training program away from the caregiving site, participants are better assured of uninterrupted time. Other caregivers are then allocated the responsibilities of the person attending the workshop. In summary, make the workshop location comfortable, useful, private, and away from active work situations!

Leadership

The ideal leader of a grief education workshop is a caregiver, a counselor, and an educator. All three skill dimensions are needed in each workshop. In addition, the leader must be comfortable with a group format. This includes experience in a variety of styles of leadership and having a sense of how a group functions. Grief education using the workshop model is group work, even though the group life may be very time limited.

Grief education (group work) is both cost-effective and therapeutically indicated. It is more efficient to work with caregivers because they can then better assist elderly persons who are facing loss, grief, and death. The elderly population, because of its growth and needs, can consume much time and resources. This can be quite overwhelming to trained and untrained personnel.

Second, workshops are indicated because of the supportive nature of groups. This is evidenced in the following ways: The group provides norms that can help inexperienced and frustrated caregivers. It builds structure and sets limits on an individual's capacity to regress to needy states. Also, in a group setting, participants see one another in various stages of grief and recovery. Learning occurs before, during, and after the workshop. This provides a linkage for learning in and outside of the workshop experience. The workshop format also makes coleadership possible. Shared leadership enables male and female input, specialization, the possibility of an observer role, and a way to debrief and deal with countertransference and other issues that tend to occur. Finally, the group can generate topics so that a menu of needs and interests are available to participants and leaders.

In addition to being skilled in leading group work, the leaders must take a multimodal approach, remain open-minded, and have an eclectic outlook because inexperienced caregivers and leaders often work from one perspective. For example, if a leader has an affective bias, he or she may be overwhelmed by feelings. In the field of grief and loss therapy, this can feel like getting in touch with Mount Saint Helens. If, on the other hand, a cognitive approach is taken, an individual may engage in useless intellectualizing, which is equivalent to shuffling chairs on the Titanic.

Leaders must be flexible and able to work in different directions. One way to remember this is to think of the ideal grief educator as a leader knowing and working with the basics at all times. This means the leader will consider the many conceptual and experimental dimensions of the material as well as the individual. BASICS is an acronym that is useful for describing this concept and process. When a leader works with basics he or she is paying attention to the following domains:

B ehavioral
A ffective
S omatic
I nterpersonal
C ognitive
S piritual

Finally, leaders of grief education workshops for caregivers of the elderly must have experience with aging (aged) people going through grief and loss. A leader must be developmentally oriented and value the final stage of life and the universal and unique experiences of aging, grieving, and dying. To value old age, he or she must also know about other stages of development and normative grief processes in those stages.

This means that the grief educator must not be burned-out, bitter, condescending, or otherwise negatively biased toward elderly or grieving persons. That is to say, the best leader is one who has known and liked an aged and grieving person!

In my case, this person was my dad! At age seventy-five, my dad called everyone in the family to come and say good-bye just before he underwent a triple bypass operation. He even called his estranged brother. He made it through the operation and returned home. One year later, he was out in the stream behind his house fishing. He was stumbling and falling, but nevertheless fishing, as he had for seventy years. He died the day after such a fishing expedition. He fell face forward on the floor and died immediately. It was he who had declared after the last operation a year previously, "I have to live my life the way I want to live it. If I have another heart attack, I want it to be the big one."

When I try to identify with aging persons and the freedom they need to control their lives, the good and perhaps not so good choices they make, I think of my dad, and I focus on the uniqueness of each person's life and dying.

Format

Ideally, a grief and loss workshop should run about twelve hours. This could be a weekend program, a two-day program, or a six-week format of two-hour sessions. Some follow-up is important for working with experiences that occur after the initial contact with the material. However, in designing a training program, there will always be participant and time limitations. Therefore, it is important to remain flexible in designing educational opportunities.

The following formats have proven successful:

- A one-day workshop (six hours)
- A one-day workshop with follow-up one month later (eight hours)
- A two-hour in-service program (on each of three work shifts)
- A two-hour orientation for new employees

Success in any one of these formats seems to depend on the ability to clarify goals and adapt the workshop design in a manageable way. It is crucial to know what outcome is desired and to formulate objectives with the format and time factor in mind.

For example, the one-day workshop with follow-up one month later is my favorite design. Reductions and reallocation of staff, priorities, available space, as well as other factors may make this a difficult format for some situations. Admittedly, two-hour workshops are fast becoming the program of choice. This brief in-service session is somewhat offset (in effectiveness) by staff attending more than once, inclusion of slightly different material, and provision of a variety of other workshop experiences.

PHASES OF WORKSHOP DESIGN

In designing a workshop to meet your needs, you will want first to establish your mission. Second, you will want to set forth your goals and objectives. Third, you will want to determine how participants get into your workshop. Finally, you will need to develop an evaluative instrument to determine the degree to which you have achieved your goals and objectives.

Establishing a Mission

Immediately following the recognition of need and desire to engage in grief education, it is important to establish a mission. By establishing a mission, you will be determining the reason for doing grief education in the first place. You will want to write down what it is you think you want to do, before you do anything else. Chapter 1 of this book is a good review, as it provides a rationale for grief education. This may be a helpful starting place, but you will want to decide on specifics for your unique situation. Establishing a mission statement will provide energy and meaning to your endeavors. In most cases, the mission is the provision of improved care for elderly persons through the education of caregivers about aging, grief, and loss.

Setting Goals and Objectives

If improved care is a mission, then grief education for caregivers is the goal. Remember, it is wise to set goals that can produce specific objectives (see Chapter 1). A goal is a desired outcome, and it is possible to have a number of goals.

Objectives are the small steps (minigoals) by which you obtain your overall goal. Often objectives are worded in the form of actions to take. You may have general objectives for grief education, as in Chapter 1, and you may have objectives for individual sessions and participants. There are both program and participant goals and objectives. It is important to know something about establishing measurable goals and objectives for each workshop and for the educational program as a whole. To summarize, you will want to know what your outcome is, how you intend to achieve this outcome, and how you will know if you have done so.

Getting Participants into the Program

This part of the workshop design involves considerations about those persons who are the focus of your workshop. It is essential to decide who will be invited to attend. How will these persons be empowered, or encouraged, to come to the program? Questions of authority and empowerment, both personal and administrative, will need to be part of the workshop design. Highly motivated participants are essential.

Motivation is both a systemic and a personal factor of workshop design that must be addressed in the early phase. It is a good idea to work with the whole system, building a foundation with the administration, the educational department, the pastoral services department, and each individual discipline.

Evaluating the Program

When beginning workshop design, it is essential to develop an assessment instrument. This may be informal or formal. A formal one is most helpful and is most frequently accomplished through a closing evaluation. Informal evaluations are accomplished by encouraging participant feedback during the workshop and in other settings. Informal feedback can provide a general measure of the success of workshops given over time. It does not give a reliable individual or specific workshop measure. The best approach is to have a brief form that can be collated and that is helpful to the leaders and to future program design.

GENERALIZATIONS OF LEARNING

Grief education workshops have lives of their own. They have a beginning, middle, and ending. They are evaluated and restructured over a period of time. After a number of programs and a number of years, a specific format develops that, with continued evaluation, can be called "your program." The process of design, implementation, and review of this program can lead to understandings that can be generalized to future efforts and other situations. The following generalizations, often learned by trial and error, are essential to a sound educational program:

Measurable goals and outcomes. This has been discussed previously. Refinement and changes of evaluative formats are a good idea. Well-formed evaluations produce meaningful goals and outcomes in the future. Think of this complete process as a quality improvement measure!

A way to involve the whole facility, family, ward, and unit. It is helpful if the workshops are publicized and discussed regularly. Often, specific situations demonstrate the need for caregivers to have grief education in order to be more aware of the special needs of the elderly. It is helpful if these needs are identified in the general operations of the ward, unit or family.

A way to diffuse emotions, and struggles, and to provide feedback. Grief education will evoke feelings among the participants. It is wise to acknowledge this at the very beginning of the workshop. Caregivers respond more openly to the goal of providing better care for the older person through increased insight, skill, and understanding of self and client.

A way to deal with participant expectations. It is helpful to have participants share their expectations, problems, concerns, and focuses at the beginning of the workshop. These are recorded and posted. An attempt is made to include these in the program as appropriate. Expectations that are not possible to meet during the workshop may be placed on a "parking lot" sheet (large newsprint on a wall) to be met in other ways.

A resource network. It is essential that leaders be available to participants. The nature of this availability and of other resources should be clearly stated at the beginning of the workshop and re-stated at the end.

SUMMARY: THE TEN COMMANDMENTS OF GRIEF EDUCATION

I once attended a hospital's grand rounds program, during which Dr. Tom Fox (1989) discussed the "Ten Commandments of Working with Borderlines in an Outpatient Program." The following generalizations are adaptations of this idea, with a changed focus on grief education:

1. Thou shalt hold no faults or easy answers.
2. Thou shalt monitor thine own pulse.
3. Thou shalt establish clear educational goals and turn to them often.
4. Thou shalt think developmentally.
5. Thou shalt honor thy participant's, patient's, resident's, and own strengths and cognitively restructure their weaknesses in pursuit of their strengths.
6. Thou shalt restructure and adapt supportively.
7. Thou shalt think eclectically and read constantly.
8. Thou shalt know thy limits lest you smash upon them.
9. Thou shalt get help when you need it and do not feel guilty about it.
10. Thou shalt show enlightened self-interest to care for yourself, work with a co-leader, and avoid burnout.

By working in the field of grief education, one will eventually be able to affirm what is really important about caregiving, bereavement, and working with the elderly. One also learns to take risks. In this field, risk taking is an essential part of the role of leadership because needs often appear so rapidly that caregiver responses must be quick, unrehearsed, authentic, and timely. They also must be individualized. Workshops on grief, death and dying, and elderly people help many persons who are taking the workshop, or seminar, respond well even when they themselves are grieving. In this sense, the ability to reach out, to risk being there, and doing or not doing something is a much-needed capacity for caregivers to develop.

Another essential of leadership and caregiving is enlarging one's capacity to trust. One has to trust that grief is a natural process, that most people complete it, and that there are ways to help grieving persons. Affirming what is important, taking risks with people, and trusting the process are three important lessons gleaned directly from grief education experiences.

Chapter 6

Caregivers: Practitioners, Helpers, and Companions

In previous chapters, we have focused on grief education—what it is conceptually and what it looks like in a workshop format. We have also looked at the aging person and grown in awareness of some of the developmental issues and challenges that are faced in old age, such as loss, grieving, and death. In this chapter, the role of persons who help care for the elderly will be discussed in greater depth.

In thinking about the caregiver, several questions come to mind: Who is a caregiver? What does a caregiver do? How and where does this caregiving take place? What are the problems faced by caregivers? How can caregivers be assisted in minimizing these problems and in improving their services? These are some of the questions considered in this chapter.

WHO IS A CAREGIVER?

Caregivers can be family members, friends, a community, religious persons, and medical personnel (including nurses and nursing assistants) and other professional persons. Due to the diversity and the complexity of roles for individual caregivers, it is important to have as broad a definition of caregiver as is possible. When the definition of caregiver is too narrow, services are usually not as comprehensive or of as high quality as would otherwise be possible. The confusion of which caregiving personnel are involved or could be involved in the meeting of the needs of individual elderly persons leads to limited resources, potential overlapping of some services, and omission of some very basic needs. Broad, but clear, definitions of caregivers and their services can provide for improved services, less conflictual events and relationships, and more energy for the persons providing the care. In this light, the following definition may be helpful:

> A caregiver is one who by choice, through delegation, or by training and job description, assists in helping individuals in meeting their needs.

DEVELOPING A CONTINUUM OF CARE MODEL

There was a time when elderly people were encouraged to meet their own personal needs and to rely on others only as a last resort. Hence, they would stay in their house, or apartment, or even on the street for as long as they could. Only after much personal agony, crisis, or observation by a caring person that important needs were not being met would the elderly person be the object of problem solving about what could be done to improve his or her lot. Responses during these times were crisis reactions that often led to caregivers feeling pressured and resistant to doing what needed to be done or even investigating possible options. It was considered a horrible event for an elderly person to move in with family, to move to a retirement community, or, heaven forbid, go into a nursing home.

The unique needs of elderly and dying elderly persons require that the role of caregiver be redefined to include services in the home, in outpatient settings, in retirement communities where meals, nursing, activities, and other services are available as needed, and in long-term care facilities. This way of viewing changes in the lives, abilities, and needs of elderly people make this continuum of care model a very supportive approach that is open to innovative services. It provides functions for caregivers that change as the individual changes. The continuum of care model is shown in Figure 6.1.

Note that the core of care resides in the elderly person because the life being lived belongs to the individual at all times. This is called *self-care*. The use of caregivers is based on clearly assessed

FIGURE 6.1. Continuum of Care Levels

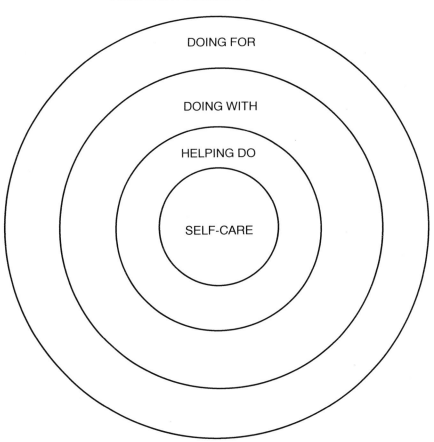

or requested needs, which, in optimal situations, are planned for before that need occurs.

The first shift in a care level usually occurs when the person realizes that he or she needs help doing the things normally accomplished alone. The role of the caregiver at this stage is called *helping do*. This may mean helping clean storm windows, bringing in meals-on-wheels or other services, and maybe giving the person a ride to church or elsewhere. The need is usually identified by the elderly person, although occasionally family members notice that some things are not getting done.

The next stage of caregiving services are described as *doing with.* Individuals find they require more help, and caregivers may be needed to help with reading and writing letters, clothes fastening, getting up and down stairs, and making sure medications are taken in appropriate and prescribed ways.

There are times when individuals need a lot of *doing for.* This time may come slowly or as a seemingly quick shift in the individual's level of need. As these shifts in care occur, the roles and responsibilities of caregivers become greater and greater.

By using the continuum of care model, the caregiver's focus can begin, end, or carry on whatever the living context of the elderly person is, whether at home or in a hospital, nursing home, retirement community, or other independent and assisted-care programs.

CONTINUUM OF CARE CONTEXTS

In our society today, most elderly persons live in a home or apartment. They may not live independently, however. Some live alone; some share their space with a spouse or roommate; and some live with their adult children in the family's living quarters or in a connected apartment. A growing number of aging persons move into a retirement community or an assisted-living arrangement in their middle-old years. About 5 percent of the elderly population live in long-term care facilities, such as hospitals, assisted-care homes, or nursing homes, depending on the degree of medical care or assistance needed.

Four examples of caregiving contexts are being provided here to illustrate several environments in which elderly persons may live at the time of their deaths. These examples describe the varieties of caregiving roles and grieving issues involved for the dying, the bereaved, and the caregiver, who may also be grieving. The first is the story of a young-old woman dying at home. The second is the story of a middle-old man dying in a general hospital. The third example is a composite view of an old-old woman dying in a long-term health care facility. This is followed by a poem written in a similar context some twenty-two years later.

Example 1: Dying at Home

It was during the fall when it became evident that her health was becoming increasingly worse. She was seventy years old and living with her husband in their own home, which she had decorated, cleaned, and cooked in for some time. She now spent much of her time in her own bedroom; her husband moved into another room so as to get some sleep and to allow the other room to be arranged to meet her needs. From her window, she could see the remnants of last year's garden. Now, as winter held way, she hoped to see one more flower and to have one more family Easter at the church in town. Her children visited her frequently during the final months. She needed shots to ease some of her pain so her daughter, a nurse, stayed with her to provide what help she could. Easter came and all was done as the mother wanted it. Yet, swallowing became more difficult for her. She required closer supervision than the daughter and father could provide. Hospice was asked for help, and they took some of the burden off the immediate family's shoulders. Family members who were not able to be present much of the time came and did what they could as often as they could. She died in her own home.

Example 2: Dying in a General Hospital

He was seventy-five, going on seventy-six, when he had a heart attack. He was rushed to a hospital some twenty minutes away. He had chosen the hospital because of its religious name. He, himself, was not Catholic, but he liked having the nuns go by his window in intensive care. It gave him hope and companionship. At first, they thought he would die soon. His bed could be seen from the nursing station, and nurses entered his room every few minutes. They were caring, friendly, and efficient and in a brief number of hours got to know something of his personality. Eight members of the family waited throughout the evening and the next day. The doctor asked the family to choose a spokesperson and said he would only meet with that person. The rest of the family waited for news. They were allowed to visit with him (a husband, grandpa, and dad) only once an hour for three minutes. This was frustrating for him, and the family. Nevertheless, all members of the extended family were able to see him, and he made a point of saying good-bye even as he tried to be hopeful. Two days later, he was flown some eighty miles away to another hospital where he underwent bypass heart surgery. It was painful. His recovery was good for one year and then he had another attack, falling to the floor in his bedroom doorway. His wife, who was blind, was asleep in the bed nearby and did not hear or see the fall. A grandchild, who stayed during the evening hours, found him. He was rushed by ambulance to the hospital where he was pronounced dead. The family was called the next day and asked to remove the body from the hospital as soon as possible.

Example 3: Dying in a State Hospital, Circa 1968

Lina lives on this ward. She used to live elsewhere. Once she was younger and lived in her own home. Now she and everyone else on the ward are getting much older. Like the others, she is chronically ill, suffers from limited mobility, and is unable to care for herself. She is quite senile.

Looking around the ward, one does not see many staff. Lina's care is largely custodial, focusing on her physical needs of food, clothing, and shelter. Most medical treatment and nursing care are aimed at slowing deterioration, prolonging her life, and keeping her reasonably comfortable. The critical list is reserved for those patients who are nearing death. The workload for staff is high and keeps increasing.

Dying in this place is slow and appears timeless. Often one will hear staff and families reasoning aloud about it being time for the person to die. Some patients are more likeable, and some are more disagreeable. Staff are more attached to some patients than to others. Staff are neither close nor distant with Lina.

As Lina lies dying, she has little to say about what is going on, especially in the later phases. She is isolated by being moved to another room where the curtain is closed around her. There is often limited time with family and friends. Lina's family no longer comes. Most no longer exist. She receives brief occasional visits from the clergy, who may offer a quick prayer, an anointing, or an occasional blessing. The room is often dim, with the shades drawn and the lights low.

Lina's death, when it comes, is not likely to produce highly emotional scenes from staff or peers. As could be said of many others, "In effect, then, these patients drift out of the world, almost like imperceptible melting snowflakes" (Glaser and Strauss, 1968, p. 64).

Example 4: A State Psychiatric Nursing Home, Today

In this example, caregivers come and go, as do other patients/ residents, to see this elderly woman in her late seventies. Staff make it a point of not leaving her alone, as she is in her last phase of cancer and they are unable to relieve much of her pain or fears. A chaplain is called to sit with her and another to give her an Anointing of the Sick. She is in a private room, her own room, where there are some pictures of her on the wall and a few items she cherishes about the room. Staff are frustrated about her pain level and her physical deterioration, yet they remain determined to do what they can do, and much of that means sitting nearby to provide company and assistance as needed. This goes on for a number of weeks.

Her death is quiet. Yet, she is surrounded by a couple of her favorite nursing assistants, who hold her hand as she takes her last breath. They have placed an angel pin on her shoulder. Those who have cared for her for many years now draw the curtain and wash her body, as tears slide down their cheeks. A memorial service is held several days later on the unit, and a picture is displayed for staff and residents. Everyone who is able, shares a story or memory. Some of the stories are funny, some are sad, and many are told with reverence.

Of Life and Independence

We couldn't believe
she lived so long
there was nothing
but skin and bones.
And still she lived
and fed herself
and always said,
"I love you."

Her hair stood out,
there wasn't much,
and those big brown eyes
were bulging.
She whispered now
and was alone a lot
but still she said,
"I love you."

We learned so much
and were amazed
at what she gave to us,
a will to live,
a fear of death,
a part of who she was.

CAREGIVER FRUSTRATIONS

It is impossible to work with elderly and dying persons without feeling concern about the quality of their lives and the quality of care they are receiving. Often, this frustration will be projected outward, as in the following poem based on a discussion among hospital employees, a chaplain, and a funeral director concerning a state burial for an elderly woman. In this case, it is the funeral director who is having difficulty with a state burial. His comments bring tears of anger and frustration from an already vulnerable but committed group of caregivers.

It Isn't Right

A couple of dollars
won't go far
when it comes to clothes
and things.
Certainly wood and
flowers these days
are out of this world
to pay.

For how can we leave
her there
in a simple box by the
creek.
Surrounded by birds,
and new-mown hay,
and stones that have
long since sunk.

For she should have
arrangements,
and air conditioning,
rather than
the yellow
sun.
And furthermore
she ought to have
no water,
and a bright green turf,
when at last her day is done.

So,
It isn't right
for folk to gather
and see her lying there,
with dirt so brown,
and just a few
finally left to care.

Respect is what it's all about
and we thought we were
doing that.
For we gathered round,
and wished her well,
and let it go at that.

"Still," he said, in
his dark, pressed suit,
with his wheels and

mind on a run.
"It isn't right."
She should have this,
and
she should have that,
when at last her day is done.

OBSTACLES TO CAREGIVING

External and environmental obstacles to caregiving are common in family, hospital, and long-term care contexts. It is an understated truth that elderly persons don't always want, or need, the kind of interventions offered or foisted upon them. Family, friends, and other interested persons have agendas of their own that may, or may not, match the elderly person's needs or wishes or those of the primary caregiver(s). Also, the environmental context for caring for elderly persons may not be conducive to meeting individual needs to the degree desired by the person or the caregiver. Yet, even with these and other considerations, it remains the responsibility of a caregiver (particularly one delegated with such authority and responsibility) to provide quality care for the elderly person.

Caregivers also face numerous internal obstacles. Four common obstacles in working with elderly persons are:

- inexperience,
- lack of training,
- avoidance, and
- equation of program with personal service.

Caregivers are often inexperienced in assisting dying elderly persons. In the case of familial caregivers, there may have been little or no modeling for this type of care. This is particularly true in the past fifty years or so, as societal changes have meant more delegation of care to medically trained persons. It is also true that elderly persons tend to live alone or in conditions other than with a nuclear family. This leaves less opportunity for intergenerational modeling about caregiving as a familial role. Consequently, when these individuals enter a caregiving profession, there is likely to be less personal experience available to the caregiver to use as a resource for what needs to be accomplished.

Another obstacle to caregiving is the lack of training the professional caregiver receives, both in academic institutions and in continuing education. In the past, there has been insufficient training in the area of aging populations, grief education, and care for the dying. The health care profession is just beginning to recognize these training deficiencies. In the late 1960s, it was a joke in ministerial programs that after three or four years of training the seminary would set aside one day prior to graduation to talk about how to do a funeral! It is still apparent that most health care professionals have the minimum of one course, or one portion of a lecture, on the stages of death and dying. Psychiatric students studying for certification tests have practice manuals with one or two paragraphs or questions about grief. Yet knowledge and practice are essential to good caregiving, and many caregivers are not adequately trained. As training is provided, caregivers will become better qualified to help elderly persons meet their needs.

A third obstacle to caregiving is an emotional one. Caregivers may be grieving while they are caring for others. Many caregivers, and their supervisors, do not believe it is okay to grieve openly. Frequently, a caregiver's response, if holding this belief, may be emotional avoidance when faced with the loss of elderly persons or with death in general. There are idiosyncratic reasons for this, usually found in the experiences and developmental issues of the caregiver. There are also typical avoidance reactions common for many caregivers. Aging persons remind younger caregivers that they, too, will grow old and have to struggle with physiological, psychological, social, interpersonal, and spiritual issues. They, too, will someday face death. Denial and avoidance are typical reactions, which, combined with general stress, overwork, and lack of experience and training, make for overwhelmed and underresourced individuals who have difficulty doing their job.

A fourth obstacle to caregiving is the tendency to equate program or patient care plans with the meeting of personal needs of the elderly individual. Even families will assume that having a nurse come in, and someone to clean the house or get the person to church, will take care of mom's, dad's, grandpa's, or auntie's situation. This is the externalized form of internal denial, and it is a trap, particularly in a society that is based on the get-up-and-go of youth and industry. Part of the problem is that caregivers do not know what elderly persons are like, and elderly persons may not know what is expected of them. Also, families and facilities are systems that have a role for everybody, and they become disconcerted when an individual does not fit that role. Although it is important for families, hospitals, and homes to have a general service delivery system (a way of planning for the general care of its individuals), it is essential to remember that this is a group plan that will meet some individual needs and not others. It is overwhelming for caregivers to feel that they should, or even can, meet all the needs of an elderly and/or dying person. That is not possible. However, it is important to help the elderly person, and caregivers should devise a plan that will meet as many needs as possible for that person. This will be a personal plan, not an activity or maintenance program.

TO HELP OR NOT TO HELP?

Considering the role and the obstacles and frustrations of being a caregiver, it is not surprising that many become stuck in expectations and duties without time, resources, or sufficient training and insight to meet the challenges they face. Some caregivers tend to forget that caregiving interventions consist of multiple decisions about when, where, and how to assist people. During any given day, a caregiver is likely to ask himself or herself questions such as:

- What needs to be done?
- When does it need to be done?
- How?
- Why?
- Do I want to do it?
- Am I able to do what needs to be done?

These questions are an important part of assessing each situation. This assessment often becomes an unconscious process, and it is the unconscious nature of these decisions that may cause problems, particularly if the routine is broken or decisions are questioned. Quality care and qualified caregivers depend on a heightened awareness of the assessment process. Every care assessment must include the question of desire and capacity to assist, from the perspective of caregiving resources.

The decision about whether one is the right person and is motivated to intervene is often the most frequently overlooked component in the assessment process. The predisposition to assist, to be a caregiver, must be based on solid internal realities as well as on external pressures and roles.

PREDISPOSITION TO ASSIST
AGING AND DYING ELDERLY PERSONS

The following four components are internal dispositions essential for caregivers of aging and dying elderly persons. These are not intended to include skill competencies or job descriptions but rather the personal resources necessary for good caregiving.

The caregiver who wishes to assist must:

- *have knowledge of his or her feelings regarding death.* These feelings may or may not be shared with the elderly persons, but they are essential to the caregiver's capacity to give aid. Feelings that are particularly negative must be addressed to avoid interference with caregiving.
- *be committed to the process of resolving and reviewing his or her experiences of loss, grief, and resultant concerns.* This commitment will be an extensive one, requiring time and energy and perhaps outside resources. It also will be revisited from time to time, as commitment is not a stationary state; it changes, even daily.
- *have his or her own belief system.* It is essential that caregivers come to terms with what they believe about life, aging, death, and the end of life. It is also important to know what one believes about what may or may not occur after death. Again, this may or may not be shared, but it is foremost on the minds and in the hearts of aging and dying persons. What a caregiver believes affects how he or she helps, or hinders, the elderly person.
- *know how he or she feels about aging people and like them.* It is amazing to discover that many caregivers of the elderly do

not know much about aging, have not had much contact with aging persons, and more amazingly, do not appear to even like them. It is no surprise that elderly people sense this and that it complicates their life and their dying. Usually, with training, experience, and support, a caregiver can examine his or her feelings about old people and come to feel differently. Often, reflections about an elderly person in the caregiver's family, someone who is liked (regardless of weaknesses and problems), will assist the caregiver in overcoming "agistic" biases.

GENERAL CAREGIVING INTERVENTION GOALS

Once an assessment of the elderly individual's needs and the caregiver's capacity to help have been made, the establishment of caregiving goals must follow. When working with acute grief reactions of elderly persons and with dying processes, there are four intervention goals appropriate to most situations:

- offer support by listening.
- provide opportunities to express personal perspectives.
- provide practical help.
- encourage life review.

Support is the first goal of caregiving. In both dying and grieving situations, the elderly person is to be listened to and made to feel as secure and safe as possible. Support in the counseling sense involves listening and helping the individual clarify feelings and experiences. Listening takes precedence in all phases.

The second goal is related to the first. The elderly person is to be given ample opportunity to formulate and express his or her perspective on what is going on with him or her. It is this perspective that will provide the individual with energy and meaning. It must be experienced internally. In cases in which the individual ego (self-image) may be too fragile, distorted, or fragmented (because of the present crisis, illness, or personality development), the caregiver can choose to support the individual by modeling one or more perspectives that may be appropriate. Elderly persons appear to benefit from this modeling of perspective, particularly when the caregiver is someone closer to his or her own age.

A third goal is that of being helpful in a practical sense. During the dying process, and during the grief stage of shock and denial, the elderly person will have moments when he or she needs caregivers to be helpful in concrete ways.

In the case of the dying person, letters need to be written and people contacted. Arrangements have to be made. Medication may have to be administered to ease pain. A swab or washcloth may be needed. Hands may need to be held, songs sung, and scripture read. A quiet presence may be just the right thing also. This is where it is essential to be aware of the dying process in general—what happens and what helps.

In the case of the grieving person, during the acute stages of loss, there are practical things that must be done and are of utmost importance. The bereaved may need to be taught how to proceed with rituals and with personal life. He or she may need help with meals and daily chores. A call or a visit may be helpful, as may transportation and help with notifying relatives and friends. In the early stages, practical help is essential. It must be offered or gently provided, as the bereaved may not be able or willing to ask for it.

The fourth goal is that of life review. This is always an appropriate goal for elderly persons, as it is the primary task of old age to find ultimate meaning through the summing up of one's life. It is also an essential component of grief reorganization and recovery. Life review is often an informal process. Elderly persons appear to be naturally willing to do this task, at their own speed and in their own way. Sometimes caregivers who are not immediate family can be helpful. A life review involves recognition of one's hopes, failures, and personal meaning. Sometimes this process is painful, and families may be too vulnerable to be helpful. It is important that the life review be an integrating enterprise so it should occur at the proper time in the most natural setting. Caregivers can be especially helpful here.

STAGE-APPROPRIATE OBJECTIVES

Grief education for caregivers of elderly persons focuses on the elderly person and the grieving processes, including the perspectives of the dying individual, the bereaved, and the caregiver. Figure

B (see Appendixes, Workshop 2) consists of a chart showing the tasks facing the dying person and those facing his or her caregiver.

A second chart (see Appendixes, Workshop 3, Figure E) describes phases of bereavement and interventions appropriate to each phase a person goes through when grieving. These interventions focus on physiological, psychological, sociological, and spiritual dimensions. The grief response for the bereaved and the caregiver-bereaved depend on factors of closeness and involvement.

THE ROLE OF THE GRIEF COUNSELOR

There are times when a specialist should be called in to provide counseling. The grief counselor is a fairly recent phenomenon so many counselors view grief counseling as only a small part of their practice. However, in large health care facilities and organizations such as Hospice, the number of situations requiring specialized help are recognized, as is the need for qualified grief counselors. However, most grieving persons do not seek professional help; most people manage to use personal resources. But what of those who seek and need counseling? What can be expected of a grief counselor?

In general, the grief counselor should have the qualifications of a caregiver. He or she should have training in aging, grief and bereavement processes. He or she should also have working knowledge of general counseling concepts and approaches. He or she should be able to counsel (or provide referral to someone who can) from a variety of theoretical frameworks, the most common being behavioral, pastoral, psychodynamic, cognitive, family systems, and crisis intervention. Each framework has its own methodology and strength, but all must help the elderly person move toward recovery and acceptance of reality.

Grief counseling usually focuses on one or more of the following:

- Crisis intervention
- Facilitating uncomplicated grief
- Therapy for unresolved or complicated grief reactions

Crisis intervention, as a counseling modality, involves one to six sessions to relieve immediate incapacitation incurred upon learning of the likelihood of personal death or as a result of having lost a significant person. This approach requires that the counseler-caregiver be able to assess the degree to which the dying or bereaved individual can cope in the immediate situation. Certain situations and specific individuals can be particularly vulnerable to crisis. Elderly men, for example, are vulnerable to suicide attempts after the death of a spouse. Traumatic death can be a factor in the need for crisis counseling, as can dying from a painful disease, such as cancer. Crisis intervention can also be helpful when there is an inadequacy of personal and social resources. This is especially so if the inadequacy could endanger life-supporting, coping skills. Assessment, relief, and referral are goals for this type of brief counseling intervention.

Most people do not need formal counseling interventions to recover from nontraumatic death or uncomplicated grief. When counseling is sought, it usually consists of a need to sort through normal processes of death, dying, and grieving. The counselor-caregiver, in these cases, is a facilitator of a process that tends to run its own course. When an individual is dying or grieving, compassion and comfort are provided first and foremost as supportive measures. Insight and review are middle phases. Confrontation is a technique reserved to gently assist those who may be stuck in grief work during the latter phase of grief, when the individual is between disorganization and reorganization phases (nearing the turning point between depression and acceptance). Confrontation may not need to be used at all by the caregiver. Self-help groups have been quite successful in cases of the loss of a child or spouse or losses due to major crises, such as traumatic illness. These groups do not seem to be as available to elderly people.

Therapy for unresolved grief may be necessary when grief is inhibited, suppressed, or absent over a period of time (much longer than one would normally suspect the process to occur). When grief is significantly distorted, suppressed, or absent, the feelings and circumstances of the loss and the relationship must be worked through. This can be a lengthy process. Developmental and personality difficulties from the past may be blocking the person's ability to experience the present grief and to move through it. Behavioral therapies have proven effective in cases of chronic grief and phobic reactions.

COUNSELING AND THE ELDERLY

Elderly persons benefit from frequent and short visits, stopping by, and "chats." They tend to be more wary of formal counseling procedures. As one man who had been referred for grief counseling said, "I wish the staff would just come by and say hello." Some elderly persons become extremely angry if it is suggested that they might benefit from counseling even when the suggestion is made in "someone to talk to" style.

Counseling for elderly persons is most likely to occur in their homes, during checkups, or in facilities in which other activities are going on simultaneously. Caregivers need to be open to counseling moments such as the following: around DNR and other advanced directives, around burial planning, during rituals, family events, and anniversaries, and during discussions of other needs, such as shelter, finances, attending church, or receiving sacraments.

Life review is a helpful process that should begin early in old age. Life review counseling, as a grieving process, can frequently be helpful during walks, rides, and spontaneous or planned moments. It seems to be true that caregivers who are willing to approach the elderly person are best able to provide grief counseling.

THE CAREGIVER AND SELF-CARE

Many caregivers come to grief education workshops to learn "how to" information, just as a cook might seek a cookbook and a foolproof recipe. By the end of a workshop, many of these caregivers begin to see that preparation and skill have both internal and external dimensions. The internal dimension of caregiving has much to do with self-care. Yet, it is hard for caregivers to be taught to care for themselves. I have found that those who master this lesson are most likely to go on to genuinely care for others.

How a caregiver takes care of himself or herself will be personal in nature. The following are guidelines that some caregivers have found helpful:

• Plan balancing activities to offset work with aging and dying persons.

- Set limits on certain difficult situations by working with peers, siblings, and colleagues—referring and/or trading off responsibilities.
- Learn relaxation techniques, exercise, and practice cognitive restructuring (thought-stopping techniques).
- Identify the persons with whom one can talk about feelings and receive a listening ear.
- Do some reality testing of one's own responses (with another qualified person).
- Go to workshops and seminars, particularly those dealing with stress, self-esteem, and grief.

Caregivers require a variety of personal and professional strategies when working with elderly and dying persons. Self-care strategies may need to change and develop and be reassessed periodically. The caregiving question, on a personal level, will include the question of self-care of the caregiver. Each caregiver must periodically ask himself or herself what he or she does to replenish the care given to others and to build that kind of caregiving into his or her own life.

In conclusion, caregivers must know who they are and who they hope to help. They must be aware of personal obstacles and strengths in their caregiving. They must use this awareness to assess the nature and extent of help they are able to provide. Intervention goals must be supportive and practical, with referral offered as necessary. Counselors, as caregivers who specialize in working with elderly people, also must be skilled in a variety of therapies and be creative in their approach to helping elderly persons who tend to have biases against formal counseling methods. Most important, caregivers must take care to replenish themselves through psychological, social, spiritual, and physical endeavors and through increased knowledge and supply of resources.

Chapter 7

Clergy As Caregivers

Grief education training, as described in this book, has focused on the training needs of caregivers within long-term health care facilities and other caregiving environments. As a grief educator, chaplain, and Director of the Department of Pastoral Services at New Hampshire Hospital, I have been able to use the fields of gerontology, grief and loss study, and pastoral care to inform my own ministry. It is this approach that is shared in this chapter on clergy as caregivers.

In focusing on pastoral care to elderly persons, and on the clergy who provide that care, I have found it helpful to have an awareness of the scriptural, religious, and social traditions of this care. It is also helpful for clergy to have an idea of pastoral care norms and to reflect on these as well as on personal experiences of training and ministry. Third, it is essential that clergy assess their strengths and limitations in this area. It is also helpful to be aware of typical problems the clerical caregiver faces in designing and implementing a ministry to elderly people. These assessments of tradition, training and experience, strengths, limitations, and problems will help clergy to define pastoral care to the elderly and to set pastoral caregiving goals and objectives that are both meaningful and manageable.

PASTORAL CARE TRADITIONS

The role of clergy as caregivers has its roots in scriptural tradition and in the church's life over the centuries. As caregivers, clergy have also been involved, in the broadest sense, in society and cultural traditions. These two areas of church and community have always been in conflict for Christian clergy. As the world has become more pluralistic and humanity has claimed more control over its own destiny, the role of clergy as caregivers has changed significantly. This change presents an urgent challenge for twenty-first century clergy to define and claim both a common and unique role as pastoral caregivers and as caregiving colleagues.

Scriptural Traditions of Pastoral Care

Some clergy wonder about the importance and need for extensive pastoral care to the elderly. Support and guidance for this wonderment can be found in Scripture. Generally, two foundations of pastoral care are found in the New Testament belief of faith being demonstrated by its fruits (seen in action) and in Jesus' teaching and modeling of caregiving.

A Faith in Action

Throughout the Bible, the two commands to honor God and to form helpful and caring relationships have been entwined in the lives of the people of God whose stories are shared in biblical text. Pastoral care has tried to maintain this connection through the encouragement of personal faith and faithful action. Whenever communities and individuals teeter to one extreme, they are encouraged to consider the other. Related to this is the notion that one's faith in God is best expressed in commitment to humanity.

Conversely, one's relationship with other people is rooted in one's faith in God. This, then, is a fundamental understanding of pastoral care and Christian living, shared by clergy, the church, and society. This leads people to expect clergy to know something about God, to have the experience of faith, and be able to translate this faith into daily living.

An example of this kind of expectation is found in the following poem. Here, the chaplain and another caregiver focus on different expectations of pastoral care. Both use scriptural foundations of relationship to God, through faith and action, as a measure of care for the elderly.

Save Them

She's always angry
At me I feel,

saying, I should do more.
Souls are dying, and are lost,
to Hell's long-burning fires.

I read the words.
I lean on rails, and sit
for hours and hours.
Hands get held
and foreheads wiped
and songs of faith
are sung.

Yet, still she feels
I should do more.
For souls not saved
are bound to be
in Hell's long-burning fires.

I cry a tear,
and sometimes more, as I
hold and touch and wait.
Absolutions and affirmations,
of God's love
are ever my words
of faith.

She fears the fires
they seem
to keep me from her.
So, I give her hugs,
and hold her near,
for those are my gifts
of faith.

Jesus the Caregiver

In the face of ultimate questions and of extreme crisis, such as those faced by elderly, dying, and grieving people, it is still most helpful for clergy to use the healing ministry of Jesus as a model of pastoral initiative and response. This model, in addition to being a basis for pastoral care, is easily understood, helpful to the current elderly population, and translatable to other caregivers.

Jesus' caregiving ministry focused on the optimum wellness of all persons. He recognized the universal human dignity of all children of God. He responded with supportive interventions that gave validity to universal and individual human needs. Although Jesus cared about all people, he took the initiative to seek out those who experienced great need. He paid particular attention to those who were lonely, shunned, and physically or emotionally ill. He also responded to the call, touch, and distress of those who came to him out of personal need or on behalf of friends and loved ones. As scripture recounts, he brought a child and an adult back to life and healed many who suffered emotionally and physically. He literally gave his own life on behalf of others. This, then, is the depth of the caregiving model we have in Jesus.

Jesus' expectations of caregivers are observable in his everyday practice of teaching, healing, and providing respect and dignity for all persons. The passing on of these expectations is clearly provided in the Sermon on the Mount, in which Jesus delegates this caregiving function to his disciples and to other followers. In the Beatitudes is a description of those who are to be recipients of our blessings, attentions, and caregiving efforts. We do not infer that these are the only people but rather that they are to receive significant attention. We are to focus on the needy in our midst. We know the needy as those who are, through life circumstances, most vulnerable. Those who are ill, who suffer, and who mourn are high on our priority list. Later on in his ministry, Jesus demonstrates how important caring for those who mourn is by asking a disciple to care for his own mother during and after his death.

COMMUNITY TRADITIONS OF PASTORAL CARE

From the beginning of church life, caring for the vulnerable in our midst became a central task of the church. This task was so essential that clergy and laypersons were trained and empowered to care for needy individuals on behalf of the whole church. It is not surprising that the pastoral care focus has been extended to people and communities at large. All of nature, according to the Genesis understanding of Creation, is under God's care. This trend, when adhered to by clergy, is part of ancient traditions in which religious persons (shamans, magicians, druids, or priests) were interpreters and caregivers for the community at large. Every event in life had spiritual significance and was brought before the medicine person, priest, or healer.

Worden (1982) correctly points out that the world today is pluralistic and that people now tend to turn to other caregivers for help. This observation does not discount the tradition for clergy to be caregivers and to be involved in the community at large. It does, however, challenge clergy to define afresh the clerical caregiving role in each generation.

PASTORAL CAREGIVING EXPERIENCES

It may be fair to suggest that congregations, and persons in society, secretly suspect that individuals are born to be clergy. This sense of destiny is perhaps fostered in the calling of the Old Testament prophets and the commissioning of the disciples of Christ. This may be so. However, an equally valid view of clergy as caregivers can be found in personality development and commitment of each individual to learn and practice pastoral caregiving. It is in this light that one finds seminarians and pastors struggling in parish, and in educational experiences, to integrate personal feelings and experiences into an understanding of self as caregiver to the elderly, grieving, and dying.

Early experiences of pastoral care and training often set the tone for lifelong ministry. Recently, I started to pay attention to the pragmatics of pastoral care that colleagues provide in this field. The attitudes toward this aspect of their ministry can be generalized, for the purpose of discussion, as two pastoral approaches:

Approach #1:
There is always something else to do besides
visit a shut-in or an old or dying person!

I have heard more than one pastor come right out and say that visiting shut-ins is a waste of pastoral time. It is amazing how low this is on many a clergyperson's list. I call this the "I would rather be golfing approach." Even though some clergy avoid visitation of shut-ins and old or dying persons, many would say that this is one of the pastor's most important tasks. The pressure to visit can lead to avoidance and guilt. For example, one minister reported, during a support group for clergy, that he had had a dream the night before in which all the older women in his parish had gotten together in heaven and said, "Oh, he didn't visit you either!"

Approach #2:
In visiting shut-ins, the hospital, or old people,
get in and out as quickly as possible!

When faced with the task of caring for the elderly, many pastors set out with the objective of spending the least amount of time possible. This can be called the "bump and run approach." All of us in the clerical profession have, I suspect, at one time or another, bowed to the pressures of duty and obligation and used this approach.

Early Ministry and Training Experiences

In looking at my own early training and pastoral experiences, two stand out in particular. The first is from a first semester Old Testament course. The second is a reflection on my early years of ministry in my first parish.

Twenty-three years ago, I enrolled in my first class at seminary. It was an Old Testament class. I was excited and frightened in equal amounts. As I reflect now, I chose to write an exegesis on the call of Isaiah (6:8). As could be expected of a first-year seminarian (who had dreamed as a little girl of becoming a missionary), I identified strongly with Isaiah's feelings of inadequacy, coupled with a probably small "Here am I! Send me." Nine years later, this same identification would be reclaimed in an ordination paper.

Continuing to reflect on my ministry to the frail elderly, I reviewed next my first parish ministry, some seventeen years ago. I remember enjoying visits to elderly persons, once I got around to it. I remember putting such visits on my list, and on my list, and on my list! Somehow, it seemed to take nothing short of an act of God or a semiannual review to get me to visit elderly shut-ins. When I did visit, people liked it and word spread that I was good at it. As I think back now, however, it was very low on the list of things I actually did.

As I reflect on these two experiences of training and ministry, I find that the feeling of inadequacy and of inability to prioritize work with elderly persons is common among clergy in general. A closer look at these two experiences shows problems of definition and of commitment. Feelings of inadequacy of response can be seen as resulting from problems of self- and role definition. The inability to give priority to this aspect of ministry can be a problem of commitment. Commitment problems, or problems of heart, are also problems of self- and role definition.

ASSESSMENT OF CLERGY AS CAREGIVERS

Problems of self- and role definition are inherent to caregiving. Each individual must struggle with his or her strengths and limitations and come to an understanding of who he or she is as a caregiver. This is usually accomplished over a period of time, through a combination of inner reflection, training, and feedback. Such a review, although remaining rooted in individual style and development, will also put the pastor in touch with common issues for clergy as caregivers. A review of this nature is likely to include some common limitations and strengths in the caregiving role.

Pastoral Limitations

The following is a list of limitations that many pastors face in grief ministry. Problems often fall in these six areas:

Seeing the whole. Many pastors have not developed a vision (conceptual and experiential) of ministry to the grieving elderly. Further, they have not related this ministry to their overall ministry and that of the church.

Education and specialization. Clergy are often limited through the lack of training in the fields of gerontology and grief and loss. This can be a lack of personal, academic, and practical training and experience.

Time restraints and priorities. Clergy, whether pastors in the parish, chaplains, or counselors, face time constraints and management issues.

Inadequate administrative planning can be a serious limitation in chronic situations, times of crisis, or uncomfortable areas of ministry.

Role specificity. Clergy have pastoral roles that they enjoy and for which they feel most qualified. The number trained to work with the aged are few, as are those who specialize in grief work. In a world in which there is an emphasis on specialization, clergy may not see grief work as ministry and may also fail to provide coverage or to delegate the role.

Feelings and stress. Clergy have personal fears and feelings about growing old, about loss, and about facing personal dying and death. There is also a great likelihood that clergy are stressed and stretched to personal limits in their ministry. These two factors can be limiting to the individual clergy and his or her work in this field.

Self-knowledge. Clergy can be limited in insight. They may not know their personal limitations and strengths. This lack of self-knowledge can lead to acting out behaviors, such as avoidance, overidentification, intellectualizing, and pontificating, with grandiose responses and impersonal answers.

Pastoral Strengths

Clergy have a number of strengths which they share in common with other caregivers and some which are unique to the clerical role and to the individual. It can be a strength for a pastor to identify these assets. The following are general clerical strengths:

Elderly people trust clergy. This is perhaps a controversial point in today's world in which clergy have received national media coverage that demonstrates the brokenness of individual clerical relationships. It is also controversial when one pays attention to polls indicating that clergy are not turned to for help as frequently as has been claimed. Nevertheless, it has been my experience that the elderly, in particular, trust clergy to be benevolently interested in them, whether or not clergy demonstrate this interest.

Clergy as provider of continuity of care. It can be considered a strength for clergy to participate in people's lives: their aging, celebrations and family rituals, illnesses, and last moments of life. In this light, clergy are primary caregivers who can be involved in many dimensions of an individual's life over the years, and they can use this experience in their helping endeavors.

Accessibility. At least in theory, the pastor's door is open. In reality, this is a strength, when the pastor carefully demonstrates the nature of his or her pastoral accessibility.

Counseling function. It is a strength for clergy to receive grief and loss education and to be able to listen and support persons facing the challenges of aging and of grief and loss. In these times, people want to know about important questions of God, faith, and living. Clergy can be invaluable in their willingness to be present with the elderly—to struggle and affirm beliefs during this stage of life and during difficult times.

Mutual reciprocity and transcendence. The give-and-take of pastoral relationships can bring meaning to the helper and the recipient. It is through this give-and-take that humanity finds relationship with self and with Creator. This is a strength that can be found in grief ministry and in working with the frail elderly.

PROBLEMS WITH THE PASTORAL CAREGIVING TASK

We now turn to what the mental health field would call service delivery problems. In the previous section, the focus was on common strengths and limitations of clergy as caregivers. A similar review can be undertaken of the caregiving task itself.

In general, clergy (as well as other caregivers) face five problems in caring for grieving and dying elderly persons. From a technical point of view, these problems could be called obstacles to caregiving. Pastoral care problems are likely to occur in these areas:

- Planning
- Troubleshooting
- Dealing with the novel
- Habitual responses
- Dangerous and technically difficult situations

Planning problems are unfortunately usually discovered during caregiving itself. It is during these moments that the lack of long- and short-term goals, strategies, and follow-up evaluation become evident. It is important to plan for this type of ministry. To do so, the pastor must understand the needs of aging persons, the effects of loss, and the process of grief. The pastor must have some skill in helping the elderly find spiritual meaning in their lives and deaths. Old age is a natural part of the life cycle; it has a place in the life of the church and in forming the ministry of the clergy. Regular planning and review of ministry to the elderly is essential.

The *lack of troubleshooting* is an equally important problem in ministry. A troubleshooter is one who is trained to be aware of possible problems in a system. Clergy must learn to anticipate problems and to consider how to handle them. In working with elderly persons, it is important to assess each individual's potential for aging and grieving complications. Each individual is unique. A caregiver needs to be flexible, with an ability to adapt and change quickly. Troubleshooting means knowing general characteristics and processes and anticipating individualized responses. Death by suicide and/or trauma, long extended dying, and the influence of dysfunctional families are all such situations that need to be considered in advance.

Dealing with the novel can be a problem for clergy, who are often conservers of tradition. In this sense, they are often able to relate to elderly persons, who also can be quite conventional in their later years. This can become a caregiving problem in light of recent sociological changes, however. Many pastors, for example, are not aware of the intricacies of advanced directives, such as living wills, do not resuscitate orders, or durable power of attorney used to carry out the wishes of the elderly during the dying process. Clergy often do not consider the possibility of remarriage of elder persons. New rituals may have to be designed to meet the needs of the unchurched, the incapacitated, and problem situations of the day. Some elderly persons do not turn to a clergyperson because they fear he or she will not be open to their expressions, experiences, and wishes. Caregivers need to keep up with new resources and relationships available to individuals.

Habitual responses can lead to planning problems. Learning ministry and pastoral care as a "how to" cookbook methodology can limit the life and energy needed in this field. The danger here is focusing on the universal at the expense of the individual. Each of these five problems has an element of relying too much on habitual response or of not having a habitual response to begin with, as in the case of planning problems. Examples of behaving by habit are found in sermons that glorify a person who was very dysfunctional. They are also found in giving permission to die to a person who wishes to remain hopeful and thereby live another ten years. Ritual responses are very important and should be taken seriously. However, when a response has no meaning, it can be at best a nuisance and at worst contribute to further pain and anguish.

Dangerous and technically difficult situations can also be a problem, when a caregiver underestimates the needs and responses of elderly persons. Some of these have been discussed earlier. They include the high rate of male suicide in the middle months of the first year of bereavement, the high rate of suicide attempts (such as not eating) by elderly males, and females who want to die. Also included are the use of life support machines, communication with emotionally and developmentally challenged persons, and the effect geographical distance has on caregiving, support, and rituals.

A DEFINITION OF PASTORAL CARE
TO THE GRIEVING AND ELDERLY

Clements (1980) gives a sound definition of pastoral care for those experiencing aging and grief. He calls the aspect of caring for the dying and the grieving *diakonia*, that is, "the implementation of faith in loving service to humanity." Certainly, what we do for the care of the frail elderly (for those who face so much change and loss of relationships, for those who face the final task of life as we know it—dying and death), we do on behalf of the church, of our own community, and for God. Those who work with the frail elderly will be the first to say that this kind of caregiving is perhaps the least sought out and the least rewarded from a cultural and social perspective. Paradoxically, as is the Christian way, the faith and energy we have in this work is therefore a recognition of meaning and of the dignity of humanity itself.

THE GOAL OF PASTORAL CAREGIVING

The goal of pastoral caregiving is to affirm the individual, his or her existence as a person and the meaning of his or her life. There are many ways to be helpful to another person. This meaning can be found in working with the person who is dying and with those who are bereaved. Pastoral caregiving to the bereaved and dying, in this sense, always focuses on the relational aspect of life. To this end, clergy, as caregivers, need to assess their motivation and capacity for help (including their own personal and professional strengths and weaknesses), the nature of the individual opportunity for ministry, and their ability to set and achieve intervention goals.

One example of this type of caregiving is found in the grief work of Pastor Dietrich Bonhoeffer, who affirmed his grandmother's life, her dying and death, and her legacy of faith and wisdom for generations to come. In a small book titled, *Meditating on the Word* (1986), Dietrich Bonhoeffer has left to succeeding generations his experience as a bereaved grandson and a caring pastor to a woman of ninety-three, his grandmother. This book includes a short homily, given by Bonhoeffer in 1936, titled "At the Funeral of Frau Julie Bonhoeffer." In this brief and powerful homily, Bonhoeffer expresses his understanding of God, his personal beliefs, and his experience of relationship with his grandmother. He concludes:

> And now we will not be sorrowful anymore. That was not her way. She never wanted to make anyone sad. We must return to our work and to our daily lives. That is the way she intended it. Above all else, she loved the deed and the day's work. We want to go forth from her grave strengthened by her life and death, strengthened much more by faith in the God who was her refuge and continues to be ours, strengthened by Jesus Christ. May the graciousness of the Lord our God be upon us; prosper the work of our hands; prosper our handiwork. Amen. (Bonhoeffer, 1986, p.71)

This clerical goal of affirmation of the individual, his or her existence, and the meaning of his or her life coincides with the general caregiving goal described by the White House Council on Aging in 1971. Here the focus is on spiritual well-being for the aging person: "Spiritual well-being is the affirmation of life in a relationship with God, self, community and environment that nurtures and celebrates wholeness" (Shelly et al., 1983, p. 19).

The concepts of well-being and care are combined in this project as wellness-care. All caregiving can be genuine efforts to provide for the total well-being or wellness of the person. This can be done only in the context of understanding all dimensions of what it means to be human. For caregivers in general, this means considering the physiological, sociological, psychological, and spiritual needs and development of people.

PASTORAL OBJECTIVES FOR WORKING WITH THE AGED, BEREAVED, AND DYING

Inexperienced and overwhelmed clergy tend to approach ministry as a provision of specific tasks in a given number of areas. The typical pastor has a number of categories of pastoral intervention based on typical pastoral roles. These usually include preaching and liturgy, ritual and sacrament (or ordinance), education, pastoral care and counseling, and community work.

When an event or need occurs, a pastor often turns to one of these areas/roles as a framework for ministry. For example, when someone dies, pastoral care may consist of a pastoral visit to the family and perhaps a prayer. A pastor may then meet with the family and discuss the rituals of a funeral, memorial, or graveside service. Sometimes, the pastor will return to the bereaved person's house after a service, and occasionally, he or she will follow up with a telephone call a week or two later.

This approach, although common, is limited. When examined more closely, it tends to fragment pastoral interventions into a series of habitual tasks. Also, it tends to focus on categories of ministry rather than the needs of the bereaved and/or dying person. Third, it focuses on a brief event rather than on the wholeness of life that encompasses many tasks, changes, and challenges. Finally, the "role" approach tends to limit opportunities for growth and change for the pastor, the church community, and the grieving person and his or her loved ones.

Another approach is to focus on the whole person in light of a variety of needs. Elderly persons need to experience ministry in a way that is helpful to them. To do this, we need to see ministry to elderly persons from a developmental viewpoint. As such, the focus would be on the normative course of old age and its issues. This would include ministry in times of loss and with the dying person. The following four examples of this style of ministry reflect the needs of elderly people, as they grow older, grieve, face their own deaths, and experience rituals of faith.

Old Age and the Meaning of Life

During old age, there is a natural tendency to review one's life and to find meaning in one's personal history and existence. A natural pastoral wonderment in relating to elderly persons would be the question of how he or she feels about his or her own life. The answer to this question reflects how a person has developed spiritually. As an elderly person talks about his or her life, a sense of meaning and purpose, a philosophy of life, begins to emerge. He or she demonstrates how he or she relates to God and/or to a higher power. Through this life-review process, the pastor will get a sense of how the individual feels in connection to nature, people, and his or her tradition. During the course of such a review, many elderly persons will be able to claim their talents and affirm themselves.

Opportunities for life review will be moments for working on the spiritual aspects of meaning in life, the psychological goal of self-individuation (ego integrity), and the sociological goal of lifestyle integration. During young-old age, the focus of life review may be on transitions and lifestyle changes. This, of course, is likely to show up at other times as well. Usually, by the time the individual has reached middle-old age, he or she is acutely aware of any unfinished business. Pastoral awareness of this will be helpful in encouraging role and relationship review. Finally, during old-old age, if not before, the individual, through meaning found in life review, will be able to trust his or her beliefs and affirm the legacies he or she has provided over the years to loved ones and community.

Pastoral care strategies during old age, perhaps more than any other time, focus on the initiative of the pastor. Initiative in this case means setting aside opportunities to listen, ask questions, talk about old age, and support and help with problem solving. Initiative also focuses on helping the individual develop and change perspectives, clarify distortions, and remember talents and benchmark occasions (such as anniversaries). The pastoral person who values the life of the elderly person and the gifts of old age will also encourage him or her to adapt to changes and to remain hopeful.

Grieving: The Loss of a Loved One

When an elderly person loses a significant person in his or her life, it is very important for the pastoral caregiver to assess how the grieving process is progressing for the bereaved. One of the best ways to begin this assessment is to gather information about the deceased. By doing so, information will accrue to provide clues as to the nature of the loss as perceived by the bereaved.

As the mourning process continues, spiritual issues emerge. A primary question at the time of any death relates to the mystery and meaning of both life and the loss. The goal of pastoral caregiving is to help the bereaved accept the reality of the loss and to move through the mourning process to affirm his or her meaning, purpose, and direction in life. This coincides with the psychological and psychosocial goals of reinvestment of emotional energy and reestablishment of social and cultural ties.

Loss of a significant relationship during old age is as painful as it is at earlier times of life. The pastoral caregiver should be aware of special issues of loss during transitions and other lifestyle changes, particularly during young-old age. During middle-old age, the bereaved is also confronted with his or her own finitude. During old-old age, the loss issue may be even more egocentric, as the bereaved struggles with his or her final days and concerns about personal comfort during the final moments of life.

During the initial stage of shock and numbness, the pastoral caregiver will want to find ways to give practical support. Certainly, the pastoral role in postdeath rituals is important. It is just as helpful to sit and listen, to pray, and to suggest resources. During the stage of dawning awareness and disorganization, the pastoral caregiver will want to accept and encourage expression of feelings. It is a good idea to listen for comments and feelings about God, faith, and meaning and to gently initiate nonthreatening conversation in these areas, if the bereaved does not do so. During the first few months, the pastor will need to continue to initiate caregiving efforts.

During reorganization and recovery, the bereaved moves on to affirm his or her life and purpose. This is a good time to continue initiating and/or following up on expressions about life, death, faith, and God. During this time, the bereaved person should also be encouraged to focus on social networks and plans for the future. Affirming of the individual's coping and capacity for choice will be more readily received once he or she has realized that he or she is able to get on with life. Due to lifestyle changes, elderly persons may need to be educated about different religious and devotional traditions at this time. This, too, can be a helpful intervention.

Personal Beliefs and Legacies of the Dying Person

When a person is dying, its is important for the individual to do the best he or she can, to believe that his or her life is of significance to God and to loved ones, and to face the uncertain future with hope. The dying person, therefore, may have the following spiritual needs:

- Affirm life and accept death
- Affirm a personal relationship to God or a higher power and see this extending into the future
- Find some perspective concerning the mystery that surrounds life, death, and future
- Feel connected to loved ones and to society through legacies and the connections of belief, and traditions

When the dying person learns that he or she is dying, it is helpful to listen and assess needs. There will be times when a dying person wants privacy and times when he or she wants to see certain people or to feel that people are nearby. He or she needs to know the facts of his or her illness and what to expect. The pastoral caregiver can listen to the elderly person and refer him or her to people who can provide information and assistance. Patience is essential as the person deals with feelings of shock and experiences periods of denial.

During the illness phase, there will likely be times when the dying individual is very angry, begins bargaining with God, is depressed, or has a wide range of emotional mood swings. It is important to listen and be aware of the pain he or she is experiencing during this time. The pastoral caregiver can be a listener, interpreter, and advocate. Elderly people usually respond favorably to conventional pastoral functions, such as communion, prayers for the sick, blessings, and confessions (formal or informal) followed by assurances of forgiveness. Many people like to talk about favorite hymns and memories of faith, family, and childhood. Clergy who know a dying person only during the final days or moments can still be of comfort by representing tradition, faith, and caring relationship.

During the final phase of life, the dying person often needs to focus internally, as he or she moves from the outer world to inner life and afterlife. This is a time for clergy to know that being present with the dying person is the essential act of loving relationship which bridges the number one fear—dying alone. The pastoral focus now is on letting the person know that there is no need to be afraid, that he or she is doing fine, that someone will be with him or her (if that is the case), and that no matter what happens God is there to love and care for him or her. Omit this affirmation about God only if you are absolutely sure the person does not believe in God or if you do not believe this to be the case. In my experience, most people want to believe in God at this time. However, the pastoral care focus is rightfully on acceptance and relationship, and that is what is spiritually important now.

Rituals and Celebration of Life

The task of the bereaved (whether individual, family, or community) is to find meaning in the deceased's life, honor him or her, and be connected to one another. Psychosocially, bereavement rituals help the grieving community recognize the reality of the loss, experience the emotional pain, and move forward in a world in which the deceased is missing. Pastoral caregivers can assist in this celebration of life by helping the elderly person and his or her family to preplan rituals that are important to them. As arrangements are made for disposal of the body and for services, the pastor can be caring in his or her respect for the faith of the deceased and in listening to the wishes of the family. Often these two are not the same. The pastor can help to further consensus and, in so doing, provide healing opportunities.

Another pastoral task may be to help individuals and the community find new rituals. J. William Worden (1982) reminds us that funeral rituals accomplish four things: make grief and loss real, help the bereaved express feelings, act as opportunities for reflection, and act as forms of social support. They are also experiences of spiritual connectedness. This connectedness of spirit is found in all five of the areas of spiritual need: a philosophy of life, an awareness of the numinous, being related to God or a higher power, being connected to nature and other people, and being self-actualized through the respecting of individual life and legacies.

Clergy can encourage people of all ages to reclaim, create, and use rituals in all aspects of life. The following are some examples of how ritual has been reframed, reclaimed, and begun anew.

Ritual Reframed

When my father-in-law died suddenly the week before Christmas, one of my first responses was, "Oh dear, this is going to ruin Christmas from now on!" My husband shared the sentiment, as did the pastor who delivered the eulogy. He, however, cleverly re-framed the problem into a meaningful ritual. During his service, he gave each member of the family a Swedish bird's nest for the Christmas tree. Dad had been Swedish, and legend said that the bird's nest, placed in the branches of a Christmas tree, was a blessing. The pastor suggested that every year when the tree was set up, we could think of Dad and know what a blessing he was to the family. It has worked just that way!

Ritual Reclaimed

A woman in her forties discovered that she had extensive cancer. She also had emotional problems and lived in a dysfunctional family. She needed something to help her in this time of personal loss and grief. Reaching back to her childhood, she remembered her roots in an orthodox Jewish family. She recalled her Sabbath Eve prayers and, through many tears, began to say those prayers daily. She did not know how many days she had left to live, but she had the experience of her faith returning to her.

Beginning New Rituals

Everyone can be encouraged to begin and practice a few small rituals. One middle-aged, developmentally challenged man who had recently lost his mother was aware that his father was getting old and that he might never go home again. When he went to his mother's graveside a year after her death, he took pictures of the countryside where he grew up and put these in a scrapbook, thus becoming the historian of his own life.

GENERAL PASTORAL CARE STRATEGIES REVIEWED

It is helpful to develop a pastoral care plan based on the needs of elderly persons. Such a plan would include general themes, spiritual needs, goals, and strategies for helping the elderly person live life fully, even unto death. Even though pastoral care strategies must always consider the needs of the individual, some suggestions, provided throughout this project, can be generalized. Seven of these general pastoral care strategies are:

- *Let people tell their story*—as much as they need to do so.
- *Encourage verbal expressions of feelings* and find ways to help nonverbal persons express their feelings.
- *Do what you can.* Be practical. Think about ordinary events and issues.
- *Be aware of theme patterns,* such as depression and faith and hope; confession and forgiveness; loneliness and God's presence and companionship; worthlessness and talents and contributions. Be willing and able to talk about these patterns.
- *Follow up on comments of meaning.* Be aware of questions and omissions about purpose, relationship to God, people, fate, and destiny. Keep pastoral input brief and simple, including beliefs and experiences that help the individual formulate his or her view.
- *Assess resources and encourage networking.* First focus on same-age peers, self-help groups, self as counselor, and then, referral for formal counseling.
- *Be a pastoral caregiver.* At all times consider yourself in a personal relationship forged from a mutual understanding of yourself as providing care on behalf of the individual, God, the church, the community, and perhaps as a surrogate family member.

THE ART OF PASTORAL CAREGIVING: LEARNINGS FROM MINISTRY WITH ELDERLY PEOPLE

Caregivers working with grief and loss, aging and elderly persons, and their caregivers can grow in definition and commitment to quality care through education, experience, self-reflection and evaluation. This is undoubtedly a demanding and sometimes painful process, but it can also be a rewarding ministry. As I look back over my own ministry, I have identified six aspects that I consider essential. I encourage other caregivers to claim their own ministry, in the uniqueness of their person, call, and experience. Here is some of what I have learned.

It is important to grieve! Set aside whatever time it takes to grieve small and not-so-small losses. Name grief and loss wherever it is found. Search your emotions (feelings and thoughts) to review the particulars of each relationship.

Plan resources. Plan ahead for times when you, as caregiver, need a caregiver. Have peers, colleagues, pastors, and/or counselors whom you know you can rely on to be a resource to you. Some people keep a journal, some pray and refer to devotionals, and some use special meditations. I cannot keep up with a journal, but I do rely on prayer, the Psalms, and on expression of feelings through the writing of personal poetry.

Try to keep up with grief and loss study. This is a huge task because the field is prolific. Do a lot of reading! Use educational training experiences as a way to review and grow in ministry.

Use the natural life review process. During old age, the phases of mourning, and spiritual searches for meaning, there is a natural tendency for individuals to engage in a life-review process. This process moves toward integration, individuation, faith renewal, and recovery. It also promotes well-being and better caregiving.

Trust your authority and integrity. I have found that the more I claim my capacity and willingness to work in grief and loss situations, the more effective and useful I become to the elderly and to caregivers, colleagues, and the community of other mental health professionals. Clergy who claim their unique persons and professional authority will be better able to help others.

Rely on grace: Accept the little kindnesses God has given each of us and look for moments of grace, in creation and in other people.

THE PASTORAL CAREGIVER
AS RECOVERED HEALER

In the study of grief and loss, there is growing emphasis on the person of the caregiving individual. This individual is expected to be a well-trained person in touch with his or her own life and issues. As a trained, self-aware person, he or she brings the goals of health, well-being, and integration to the caregiving process.

Henri Nouwen (1979) has called such a person the Wounded Healer. This image has been used in pastoral care and counseling during recent times. It does aptly describe the reality that all people grieve and that persons who are aware of their losses and their vulnerability are better able to identify with those who are experiencing pain and sorrow. However, a shifting of this image, given what we now know about grief, may be necessary. In light of grief and loss experience and study (and in light of Christ's resurrection), it might be more accurate to say that grief educators and counselors bring the presence of the Recovered Healer to the personal wounds of grief and loss. This image is appropriate for pastoral counselors and all caregivers because grief is about recovery from the wounds of life. Grief work involves undertaking a painful and searching process to come to new life. It is in healing that meaning is found, and it is in the experience of resurrection that Christ provided the meaning for life and the mystery beyond. To this end, may we all experience recovery and healing.

Chapter 8

Envisioning Eldercare:
The Next Fifty Years

Hear me, Yahweh, and be merciful!
Help me, Yahweh!
You have changed my sadness
into a joyful dance;
You have taken off my clothes of mourning
and given me garments of joy.

Psalm 30:10-11

THE FUTURE OF ELDERCARE

As we look ahead to the next fifty years of eldercare, we can expect some current problems to continue and new ones to arise. How we handle challenges presented by the complexity of eldercare needs will affect the nature and quality of old age as experienced by others, ourselves (the caregivers of today), and generations to come. The grief education training approach for caregivers of the elderly, as described in this book, has brought together theories, thoughts, and feelings about aging, grief and loss, and dying with dignity. It is the purpose of this chapter to reframe some previously identified issues by turning these into challenges and opportunities for the future.

CHALLENGE ONE:
UNDERSTANDING THE REALITIES OF OLD AGE

The realities of old age still appear to be clouded in mythology and misperception. One challenge of the next fifty years will be for researchers, caregivers, and the elderly to develop a better description of the process of aging. This description will focus on thirty-five plus potential years of living. It will describe more fully the challenges, growth, and normative developmental experiences of old age.

Specifically, we will focus our research on the phenomenon of aging. We will learn the experience of old age from the viewpoint of the elderly person. We will gain more information on the experience of direct care personnel. Future research will focus on the similarities and differences among persons who are young-old, middle-old, and old-old.

Persons over the age of sixty-five are already asking for this kind of attention to the details of aging. It will be no surprise to many of us when we begin to hear more and more from this population. They are finding their voice and we will be challenged to hear what they have to say. Just recently, a small group of elderly persons protested the lack of physicians trained in geriatric services in the state of Florida. This national news report noted that the majority of the population of this state is over age sixty-five, although the number of physicians trained in geriatric services was embarrassingly low. The reporter quoted an elderly person as declaring, "I want someone who knows how my body works at my age." This kind of information is crucial to everyone's future.

Another challenge to discovering the realities of old age will be research into the experience of the aging woman. The importance of providing better information on aging women will be crucial to understanding old age in the next fifty years. By the year 2000, there will be twice as many women as men over the age of seventy-five in the United States (Ebersole and Hess, 1990, p. 20). We must investigate further the experiences and needs of elderly women and men. We will need to know how these experiences are similar and how they are different. Interventions and helping strategies may have to change, based on this knowledge.

A third challenge of old age relates to searching for stories of how people maximize their life experiences during the later years of their lives. Suzette Hunter, in an article titled, "Adult Day Care: Promoting Quality of Life for the Elderly" (1992, p. 17), speaks to this challenge. She states, "Science has extended life expectancy, but has thus far failed to provide quality of life for those extended years. Maximizing physical, mental, and spiritual experiences during these last years is the primary goal of adult day care."

In this respect, the field is wide-open. I am reminded of a wonderful insight found in Betty Friedan's book *The Fountain of Age*. Ms. Friedan writes, "Listening to these experts on aging talk about them—the problems of those sick, helpless, senile, incontinent, childlike, dependent old people, all alone, or draining the finances of their families, a burden on the Social Security System and the hospitals—I thought how different their concerns were from those of the women and men who had been telling me about surprising changes in their own lives since they turned sixty, seventy, eighty" (Friedan, 1993, pp. 20-21). The next fifty years will be "frontier" years for all of us, as we experience living during a time in which life expectancy and quality of life are pushing the barriers of time, not just for a few people, but for many!

CHALLENGE TWO:
CREATING SPACES FOR ETHICAL DIALOGUE

Ethical quandaries are present in all life experiences. As our life span increases, so too do concerns for managing daily care issues as well as chronic care problems. In many institutions, ethical issues often relate to advanced-care directives aimed at decisions about the type of treatment an individual receives or does not receive. For example, what about breast surgery for an eighty-six-year-old with cancer? How do we feel about persons who wish to commit suicide at age seventy-two (knowing that they have a chronic and painful disease that will severely limit their life functioning)? Is there such a thing as living too long? Can the care of one individual cost too much? Can dying, with help, before "God's planned time," ever make sense? The future is here so it is not too soon to talk about ethical decision making.

The space that is needed for constructive dialogue about ethical quandaries must be large enough to involve caregivers, recipients, families and friends, institutions, and interested persons of political influence. I believe that it is more important to have this conversational space than to do things the way we usually do them. By this I am referring to a common way of making decisions—letting crisis determine the beginning or omission of ethical matters.

CHALLENGE THREE: CONSERVING RESOURCES AND ENHANCING QUALITY CARE

The future of eldercare will also depend on how well we learn to use the resources available to us. There will not be endless caregiving resources in the next fifty years. If the parallel is drawn between human resources and ecological resources, we will find that we have to provide better care with more limited resources.

A conservation of resources will necessitate more creative and holistic approaches to living during old age. Wellness care is the name I prefer to use when referring to creative and holistic approaches to eldercare. The wellness care approach is based on the principle that each individual has an optimum range of well-being and that the maintenance and extension of that range is a directive of all caregiving.

Wellness care will consist of a concerted effort to match the needs of the elderly person with available resources. Knowing that resources will not be available based on today's standards, future plans must be creatively focused. Hopefully, we will see better planning, implementation, and piloting of preventative health care and recovery programs for elderly persons. In the future, the elderly person and the caregiver will need to form a more centralized management care team, with a more clearly defined planning and review focus. Access to this system will hopefully be more egalitarian and useful for the elderly person and his or her caregivers.

CHALLENGE FOUR: USING EDUCATION AS A RESOURCE

Education is one means of conserving resources while enhancing care. The optimal future of education, as it pertains to eldercare services, will be the development of an increased sense of partnership in training functions. I envision, for example, an increased use of consumers and their families in the planning as well as implementation of educational programs for themselves and their caregivers. This will likely represent an extension of self-help approaches currently being used by other age groups. I also believe that, as the continuum of care contexts and opportunities change, educational efforts will provide valued resources because this type of education, as a rule, is based on concepts and experiences that include broad-based strategies and creative interventions.

The belief that individuals actively adjust, learn, and grow in old age will open up educational opportunities once blocked by agist stereotypes of old age as a gradual decline unto death! When old age is viewed as a period of growth marked by identifiable tasks, challenges, and opportunities, the elderly individual can be free to establish meaningful goals based on realistic personal choices. Studies of grief and loss, life span theory, and gerontology have opened the door of opportunity for the elderly and their caregivers. The grieving process can be taught and learned by the bereaved and the caregiver alike and is thus a model for the new kinds of self-help ventures that will be available to elderly persons. In the future, self-help groups which have recently become available to other adults, will become available to elderly people. These groups will be age appropriate and will help the learning and healing process through modeling and mentoring, which needs to be reclaimed for the elder population.

Education, as a resource of the future, will enable elderly persons to seek help appropriate to their specific needs. The future will probably bring a tightening of economic resources, particularly as the elderly population expands. The resources provided will, by definition, need to be more specific, more tightly organized, and subject to more rigorous accountability.

The role of the facilitator will increasingly become a more central caregiving role. This role will consist of supportive efforts, designed to meet specific needs through training, coaching, and counseling of elderly persons and their involved families, and will be collaborative in nature.

A housing model demonstrating the facilitating, or enabling, approach is the shared or assisted housing units for elderly persons who cannot live on their own for economic as well as other reasons.

Another example of this collaborative approach is found in the "shared credit" concept, wherein the elderly person volunteers to assist other elderly persons, thereby building up credit for himself or herself. This amassed credit is then redeemable to meet the volunteer's needs as they arise.

Educational efforts in the future will see a broadening of the training base for caregivers in general. Grief education has been one language used to bridge the barriers of individual caregiving disciplines. Caregivers of the future will need to know more about all dimensions of caregiving. For example, clergy, now and in the future, will need to know about the physical aspects of dying and the emotional, social, and spiritual processes. This will enable them to become more effective caregiving team members and advocates. They will need to be able to talk and listen to others, respect other caregiving disciplines, and move flexibly and confidently from an inner wisdom, training, and experience.

Caregivers will need to include themselves in the caregiving event. This means that in grief and loss, as in all caregiving, the caregiver's history and person is part of the caregiving event. How caregivers use themselves and their story is an area that is yet to be fully developed as a dimension of care for the elderly.

The observer-participant link has been suggested by many persons in the clinical counseling fields. However, it remains untapped in the field of practice. In commenting on a laboratory bereavement training program (conducted by Donovan Hommen, 1972), Merle Jordan attributed the regression observed in follow-up tests some months later to the possibility that participating clergy "were not asked during the seminar to address their own experiences of grief and loss. Since these wounded healers had not worked directly with their own pain and sadness, nor were their own personal attitudes and values regarding grief dealt with in the seminar, they had not really integrated the new information for any long-term transformation" (Jordan, 1986, p. 132).

In the future, there will be a larger number of caregivers from a variety of helping professions who will *share the language* of gerontology and grief and loss. These persons will be professionals who bring the traditions unique to their own disciplines, the insight from personal experiences, and the commitment to the well-being of the elderly person. We who are in the second, third, and fourth generation of persons trained in these fields will be the most reliable resource for enhancing the quality of life for the older person.

CHALLENGE FIVE:
CAREGIVING WHEN ALL OUR HOUSES
ARE FULL OF THE ELDERLY

In the next fifty years, Eldercare, at its best, will see society focused on healthy, happy, and spirit-filled living, as evidenced in a rich tapestry of faces and experiences. This tapestry of eldercare (which I call wellness care) will be based on the mutuality of effort of the helper and the helpee. This mutuality will be the legacy learned from the first generation of gerontologists, grief and loss researchers, and caregivers in all traditions.

I recently heard a colleague declare, "It's one thing to provide pastoral care for others. It's another thing when the care focuses on your own parents." I would add, "It is a third thing when care focuses on oneself!" I must have been thinking along these lines several years ago, when I wrote the following poem.

Eldercare and Me

I write it down as if to stay,
fifty years of eldercare I say,
what are the trends,
the movement flowing?
Looking at the future
I cannot see.
My vision grows dim
and my ears, like muffs
today, are infected.

The question becomes my own.
It's me I see at ninety-five
in a bed, or chair, much of the time.
Looking out to touch a world,
some of whom have gone before.

Me. Roles, and folks, and strings,
unraveled into a story of my mind.
Me. Now concentrating on the task of
eating, breathing. Emotions showing.

Now on task, then gone.
Back to days and times I much prefer.
What would be my own well-being?
A flower, song, a smile now offered.
A fantasy of friend remembered.
The flight of time, the salt of air,
move me past
the Thens and Nows
to timeless winds
and gentle stirrings.

Come forth a person, asking me,
"What do you need?
What then your plans
to pass the day?"

Perhaps, to remind
myself of me!
And then to sit with others.
And
if mind is fresh
and hands still nimble,
to pass communion
or say a prayer
to share a story
and visit long
with Hims and Hers
just down the hall.

In the future, there will be more and more caregivers who have struggled with personal grief and who choose to journey with others who are also grieving. There will be more and more people who know what to expect and how to help others who may get stuck in the emotions of grief. Hopefully, there will be a community of caregivers, (including the church) willing to be supportive networks for one another, in old age, in bereavement, and in life and death.

CONCLUSION

Experiences of providing grief education in a hospital setting have confirmed for me the need for persons to be trained to work with elderly persons; they must learn about caregiver grief responses and understand the effect this education has on caregiving. My experiences have also brought to light future needs, such as better descriptions of what it is to be old. Related issues just beginning to emerge come from the preponderance of women over the age of seventy-five years and the little we know about them. The management of problems related to the lengthening of our life span to ages when chronic disabilities are more prevalent is going to be an important focus. What is aging, how do women and men experience aging, and what are the costs and benefits of increased life span are all questions for the future.

The future of eldercare is likely to bring increased demand for conservation of resources, while enhancing quality of life and care for elder persons. Education, itself, is seen as a self-help tool, a way to enable the elderly person when caregiving interventions are needed and as a format for effective training in broad-based strategies and interventions.

APPENDIXES:
WORKSHOPS

Workshop 1

Attachment, Loss, and the Process of Mourning

OBJECTIVES

- Provide an opportunity for discussion concerning the theme of grief and loss.
- Increase participants' awareness of personal and professional experiences of grief and loss.
- Increase participants' awareness of some ways these experiences of grief and loss have affected caregiving experiences.
- Enable participants to distinguish between uncomplicated and complicated mourning.
- Increase the participants' awareness and potential for using a variety of resources to facilitate grief reactions as pertains to self, peers, and patients/clients.

SCHEDULE

10:00	Coffee
	Introductions
	Objectives
10:15	Personal Grief History
11:00	Lecture:
	Attachment and Loss
	Tasks of Mourning
	Phases of Bereavement
12:00	Lunch
12:30	Lecture:
	The Caregiver's Own Grief
1:30	Break
1:45	A Case Study
2:30	Closure and Evaluations

PERSONAL GRIEF HISTORY*

1. The first death I can remember was the death of:

2. My most recent loss by death was (person, time, and circumstances):

3. The most difficult death for me was:

4. Of the patients/residents I work with, the most difficult death for me would be:

5. Some of the losses I have experienced while working here that I feel I have resolved fairly well are:

6. When I think of grief and loss I find I am concerned about:

GRIEF AND LOSS CASE STUDY

Mary is a ninety-five-year-old woman who has spent approximately fifty years in an in-patient facility. During this time, she has roomed primarily with two other persons. All three residents are emotionally close.

During the past year, she has experienced some confusion. She does not remember the names of persons she has known for some time. She falls asleep during activities that normally held great interest for her. Often, when she awakens, she is disoriented and can be "grouchy." Her favorite response to a greeting is, "I'm not dead yet." She prides herself on being the last living of the twelve children in her family. Mary is quite a "faith-

---

*Adapted from Worden (1982).

ful" person and frequently declares, "If it weren't for God, we'd be nothing." She takes great joy in singing and in reciting prayers learned by heart. She also participates in sewing and other activities.

Mary's roommate, Mildred, is also in her nineties. She too is very active and involved in relationships and activities of faith and recreation. Mildred has recently expressed concerns about Mary. While she is talking of Mary, her arm reaches up and supports her head in a sorrowful manner. According to Mildred, Mary is always sleepy now, she is quick-tempered, she forgets songs and rules of games, and she is quite impatient. Mildred says this is a change from the way Mary used to be. "I try to help her," Mildred says. "I try to remind her about the rules when we are playing Hearts or about where she has put things she has lost. She doesn't like it when I remind her. We've been in the same room all these years, I hate to see her so."

During a recent staff meeting, a young woman who has worked for some time with Mary and Mildred, exclaimed, "You should see Mary now; she's giving away all her things!"

PARTICIPANT EVALUATION FORM

Please respond by circling the number on the scale that best corresponds to your opinion about each question. THANK YOU!

PROGRAM NAME: **DATE:**

	Poor			Excellent	
1. The program met the objectives that were described.	1	2	3	4	5
2. The presentation of materials was clear and well organized.	1	2	3	4	5
3. The ideas and/or techniques presented were up-to-date and relevant.	1	2	3	4	5
4. I was encouraged to share my ideas, to ask questions, and to make comments.	1	2	3	4	5
5. The instructional methods used helped me to learn the content (e.g., group discussion, exercises, demonstrations, films, slides, and handouts).	1	2	3	4	5
6. The program increased my knowledge and understanding of the subject area.	1	2	3	4	5
7. I can apply the ideas and/or techniques presented while at work. (If not, why?)	1	2	3	4	5
8. Did this instructor deliver information effectively?	1	2	3	4	5

9. Additional comments:

10. Additional programs I would like to see offered:

Workshop 2

Bereavement

SCHEDULE

9:30   Coffee
      Registrations (see Brochure)

9:40   Opening Exercise (Aging: As I Imagine Myself)

10:00 Lecture:
      Responses to Death
      Stages of Dying
      Additional Material for Advanced Workshops:
      Death and Dying Caregiving Tasks

10:45 Break

11:00 Lecture:
      Management of Grief When Working with Elderly Persons

12:00 Lunch

12:30 Lecture:
      Rituals and Beliefs

1:30   Discussion:
      Behaviors That Encourage Expression of Individual
      Needs

2:45   Closure and Evaluation

FIGURE A. Workshop 2 Brochure

REGISTRATION FORM

Bereavement

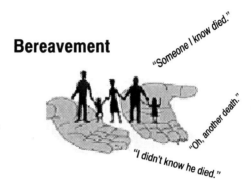

"Someone I know died."

"Oh, another death."

"I didn't know he died."

IN-SERVICE WORKSHOP #2
THURSDAY, APRIL 14, 1998
PASTORAL SERVICES DEPARTMENT
M&S BUILDING, 3 WEST

WORKSHOP OBJECTIVES

In-service workshops provided by the Pastoral Services Department and ICF/IMD Unit provide an opportunity for participants to focus on principles and practices that provide for the quality care of our elderly.

This workshop focuses on responses to death and management of grief. Helping people face the reality of death and loss frees the spirit and energy for creative living.

IF

you continue to struggle with issues of breavement, this is an opportunity to grow in this area . . .

IF

you would like some theory and the opportunity to sharpen your skills
of listening and responding . . .

IF

you have recently experienced significant loss or anticipate such a loss . . .

IF

working in the ICF/IMD Unit has caused you to be confronted with issues of death and loss . . .

THIS
WORKSHOP
IS
FOR
YOU

FIGURE A *(continued)*

SCHEDULE

9:30 a.m.
REGISTRATION AND COFFEE
A checklist on DEATH AND DYING
ATTITUDES will be completed
during this time.

9:45 a.m.
RESPONSES TO DEATH AND THE
STAGES OF GRIEVING
This presentation will focus on individual
and social responses to the potential or
real loss of someone we care for personally
and/or professionally.

AN ARTICLE: "DEATH AND DYING" WILL BE
DISTRIBUTED TO BE READ BEFORE THIS
WORKSHOP, TO BE USED TO FACILITATE
DISCUSSION.

10:00 a.m. BREAK

11:00 a.m.
MANAGEMENT OF GRIEF WHEN
WORKING WITH ELDERLY PERSONS
When working with elderly people, unique issues
of grief and its expression arise. The personal/
professional management of that grief will be
addressed.

12:00 noon LUNCH-Compliments of NHH

12:30 p.m.
RITUALS AND BELIEFS
A discussion of social and historical approaches to
death and loss is the topic. Opportunity will be provided during this part for personal and family experience.

1: 30 p.m.
BEHAVIORS THAT ENCOURAGE
THE EXPRESSION OF INDIVIDUAL
NEEDS
Participants will work in triads to role-play encourag-
ing and discouraging responses to the needs ex-
pressed by patients. The focus of this presentation is
skill attainment.

2:45 p.m.
CLOSURE AND EVALUATION

IN-SERVICE WORKSHOP #2 BEREAVEMENT

DATE OF REGISTRATION _____

BUILDING/POSITION _____

EXTENSION _____

This registration form is to be sent to the ICF Unit Educational Coordinator.
If you have any questions, please call Rev. June McCall.

AGING: AS I IMAGINE MYSELF*

CURRENT AGE:

+10

+10

+10

+10

+10

Exercise Instructions

During this exercise, you will be asked to visualize yourself aging. You may do so by writing words or phrases, by drawing yourself at each stage, or by meditating. Let us begin with the age you are now . . . and now imagine yourself as you are . . . how you look . . . what you do during the day . . . things that are important to you . . . all that is in your life as you are now . . . and now see yourself in ten years . . .

---

*After a few sets of ten, people will start commenting on the fact that they are "dead" or just can't see themselves at eighty or ninety. Continue on with the exercise until you are sure you have covered aging for all the participants. For those in their twenties, this will mean adding at least seven sets of tens.

FIGURE B. Tasks—Death and Dying

	Dying Person		Caregiver	
STAGE	**TASK**	**RIGHT**	**TASK**	**RIGHT**
SHOCK	To protect self; To prepare, alert	To react	To present accurate information	To have own response to death and dying
DEFENSE (DENIAL)	To withstand the impact of the initial diagnosis; To test the information; To buy time	To have information; To have questions answered clearly and honestly; To have hope; To not die alone; To be pain free	To be honest; To accept person's response; To formulate initial care plan; To practically assist in care of person	To have and examine relationship with dying person
EMOTIONS (ANGER)	To release emotions; To release negative emotions; To engage in existential protest; To validate "living self"	To express feelings about illness and approaching death; To be free of pain	To listen; To be empathetic; To comfort and validate person; To be a recipient of emotions	To be present; To have and express feelings; To channel feelings in helpful ways
BARGAINING	To align needs versus reality; To gain more time; To develop hope; To stall and test; To manipulate facts; To identify fears, regret, and guilt; To bring to light unfinished business; To avoid the future	To maintain hope; To participate in decisions; To make choices	To share hope; To offer choices and participation that are reality based; To talk with the person about bargains; To contract for services and relationships	To be informed and to participate; To set limits and negotiate choices and process; To maintain hope

FIGURE B *(continued)*

	Dying Person		Caregiver	
STAGE	**TASK**	**RIGHT**	**TASK**	**RIGHT**
WITH-DRAWAL (DEPRESS-ION)	To focus on self; To turn inward; To sort and (re)organize; To feel	To be treated as a living human being; To participate in decisions/control; To express feelings; To spiritually journey within; To be cared for competently and with sensitivity; To not die alone	To separate; To be sensitive to when wanted and not wanted; To foster independence; To let go; To recognize needs may be opposed	To emotionally hold the person until he or she dies; To have an inner and spiritual journey
MOVING ON (ACCEPT-ANCE)	To affirm self-image; To participate in relationship with significant others; To hope; To say good-bye; To leave	To have loved ones receive help if needed; To share spiritual concepts and experiences and to receive spiritual nurture from others; To be allowed and helped to live as normally as possible; To find meaning in the experience	To be present and to share self; To comfort and make comfortable; To find meaning in the experience; To say good-bye	To know what a good death looks like for self; To affirm the choice of the other; To say good-bye; To find own meaning in experience; To anticipate own loss and grief

BEHAVIORS THAT ENCOURAGE EXPRESSION OF NEEDS

1. Sitting by the bed or chair for a few minutes
2. Coming by to chat to see how things are
3. Inviting the person to ask questions
4. Asking how he or she feels . . . about . . .
5. Waiting for the person to respond to a question or comment
6. Accepting what the person says

7. Looking at the person and nodding understanding now and then
8. Talking about things that are important to the person
9. Responding authentically, with laughter, tears, sympathy, and empathy
10. Remembering things the person has told you about his or her life, feelings, and beliefs
11. Recognizing that the person has the right to change his or her opinions and views
12. Defining the areas of confidentiality; letting the person know what you share with others and what will be confidential
13. Respecting the individual's privacy by finding private places to talk about anything other than social pleasantries and giving you and he or she permission not to talk

BEREAVEMENT WORKSHOP EVALUATION FORM

1. TOPIC

   Was this workshop something about which you were personally/professionally concerned? Explain.

2. CONTENT

   Did you find that the content presented was/will be helpful to you now or in the future? Explain.

3. FORMAT

   Do you suggest any changes in the format of the day? Explain.

4. PARTICIPATION

   Did you feel involved in the workshop? What would have made more involvement easier for you?

5. FUTURE WORKSHOP TOPICS

   Do you have any suggestions for future workshops that Pastoral Services can give?

6. PUBLICITY/INTEREST

   What prompted your attendance at this workshop? Was it the brochure, did other staff recommend your attendance, etc.?

Workshop 3

Grief and Loss

SCHEDULE

9:00	Registration and Introductions Death and Dying: Attitudes Checklist

9:30	Lecture:
	    Hospitalization and Institutions
	    Aging and Loss

10:00	Lecture: The Dying Person and the Caregiver
10:30	Break
11:00	Lecture: Bereavement Phases
12:00	Lunch
12:30	Bereavement: The Way to Recovery
1:30	Group Discussion
2:45	Closure and Evaluation

FIGURE C. Grief and Loss Workshop Flyer

Grief and Loss Workshops

New Hampshire Hospital—Psychiatric Nursing Home Services

Spring 1990

THURSDAY, FEBRUARY 22, 1990
9:00 a.m. – 2:45 p.m.
South Function Room, Main Building

"Grief and Loss Workshop"

Including the stages of grief, complications in grieving, a developmental look at grief in the elderly years and a case presentation on anticipatory grieving issues in the Psychiatric Nursing Home Services unit.

THURSDAY, MARCH 1, 1990
9:00 a.m. – 11:00 a.m. or 1:00 p.m. – 3:00 p.m.
Yellow Room, Thayer

"Grief and Loss In-service"

An introduction to the stages of grief and complications in grieving, with a focus on resident care.

THURSDAY, MARCH 29, 1990
10:00 a.m. – 12:00 noon
Yellow Room, Thayer

"Grief Therapy"

Exploring models of grief therapy appropriate to assisting grieving needs.
How to help. When to refer!
*Note: This in-service workshop assumes knowledge
of the basic grief process.

To register, and for more program information, contact:

Rev. June McCall, extension 1234.

FIGURE D. Bereavement Phases

Levels in the Phases of Bereavement*

Phases	Biological	Emotional	Social	Spiritual
1. Shock and numbness	Tissue and cellular trauma	Feel wounded	Focus on self and personal loss	Experience of awe over loss
2. Awareness and dis-organization	Stress within body	Unorganized and/or chaotic feelings	Regression withdrawal	Disbelief, dark night of the soul
3. Reorganization	Healing	Gaining control over experience and expression of feelings	Changing self-relations	Faith, Tradition, Ritual, Belief, Restructuring
4. Recovery	Recovery of physical health and healthy functioning	Wider range, availability, and use of emotions	New/renewed sense of belonging	Experience of being part of the new creation

*See also C. Sanders (1989, p. 40).

FIGURE E. The Bereavement Process

Phases of Grief	Characteristics	Needs	Task	Caregiver Interventions
1. Shock and numbness	Sobbing; Confusion; Sorrow; Numbness; Mechanical functioning; Fleeting anger/guilt	Support; Emotional distancing; Some time alone to go through rituals	Self-protection; Stay together and go through essential tasks	Assist with specific tasks and decisions; Listen; Comfort; Hold and provide for person's privacy and as much control as he or she is able
2. Awareness and dis-organization	Yearning; Searching; Painful feelings: anger, guilt, loneliness, etc.; Behaving by habit; Sleep and appetite changes; Panic; Relying on transitional objects; Despair	To express feelings; To remember; To go about daily living	To acknowledge the loss	Encourage expression of feelings; Listen to life review; Support and reassure; Affirm reality of loss and affirm coping styles
3. Reorganization	More peaceful periods with less intense feelings and mood swings; Emerging hope and turning to future	To reenter life's mainstream; To find new meaning in life	To break emotional ties with deceased	Encourage social networking; Talk about major life themes; Encourage new coping efforts; Help with life and faith review
4. Recovery	Adapting and choosing one's own lifestyle; Moving on with hope and memory	To go about daily living; To continue with developmental tasks; To affirm one's own meaning in life	To reinvest energy in one's own present and future; Reintegration of values, beliefs, and personhood	Maintain and/or renew the relationship to its normal or negotiated give-and-take

DEATH AND DYING: ATTITUDES CHECKLIST

A Questionnaire for Caregivers

1. Age _____

2. Sex _____

3. Religion/Faith Tradition _____

4. Ethnicity _____

5. Education_____

6. Occupation_____

7. Marital/Relational Status _____

8. Children _____

9. Elderly Dependent _____

Personal Death and Dying History

10. Have you had someone close to you die? If so, describe how old you were and what that experience was like for you. (If you have had more than one experience— feel free to use another piece of paper.)

11. Describe your most positive experience having to do with death and dying.

12. Describe your most negative experience having to do with death and dying.

13. What was most helpful to you when someone close to you died/was dying?

14. Please complete this phrase: When I die I want . . .

15. Please complete this phrase: When I die I do not want . . .

16. From the following list of words, *circle all that apply* to this phrase, "When I think of dying I think of . . ."

pain	release	incomplete	alone
tears	accident	prayers	expense
old	sleep	services	food
illness	suffering	family	belongings
forever	heaven	avoid	lost
uncomfortable	parent	job	child
dark	counseling	anger	hospital

17. What other words would you add to this list?

18. When you die, what rituals would you like?

19. When you die, what ritual do you not want?

Caregiving Death and Dying History

20. When a person dies, what do you believe happens?

21. What is your role when someone you are caring for is dying?

22. What do you actually do when a patient/resident is or may be dying?

23. What is your job at this hospital? Describe what responsibilities are included in this job.

24. Which of the following interventions have you used when a patient/resident is dying? Add your own in the blank spaces provided.

Sat with the patient
Talked with the family
Talked about dying and death with patient
Helped to plan rituals after death
Remained silent and busy
Changed the sheets and other physical duties
Did my regular job/assignment
Cried with the patient
Talked with peers about the person
Called a chaplain
Brushed the patient's hair
Been speechless
Taken vital signs

_____

_____

_____

_____

_____

_____

25. As a caregiver, what I need most when a patient/resident is dying is . . .

26. As a caregiver, what I need most when a patient/resident is dead and shortly thereafter is . . .

27. I believe that healing occurs to the extent that (please finish this sentence):

28. When a patient/resident is dying or may die, what do you believe you do best?

29. When a patient/resident is dying or may die, what do you believe you do worst?

30. As a caregiver, what is most helpful to you when a patient/resident is dying or may die?

31. As a caregiver, what is least helpful to you when a patient/resident is dying or may die?

32. When was the last time a patient you worked with died?

33. How many patients with whom you have worked have died during the past year?

34. Have you had a death in the family during the last year? More than one?

Skill Attainment History

35. Have you taken a course on death and dying (grief and loss)? (Describe)

36. Please define and describe "grief."

37. What skills do you use when a patient/resident dies or may die?

38. What skills do you need when a patient/resident dies or may die?

39. Concerning the area of "grief and loss," what do you think caregivers at NHH need?

40. What could a course/workshop/support group on "grief and loss" provide for you?

Workshop 4

The Art of Caring
for the Dying Person

ABOUT THE WORKSHOP

This workshop is designed to address the complexities that dying can present to those of us who work in long-term care settings today. Issues, needs, wishes, and agendas of participants (the dying person, family, and staff) will be discussed, along with opportunities to apply prioritizing and problem solving specific case studies.

Who Is Presenting

- Social worker
- Chaplain
- Nurse

Who Should Attend

Caregivers who have participated in previous death and dying workshops or who have an introductory knowledge, understanding, and experience with grief and caring for a dying person.

SCHEDULE

8:45	Registration
9:00	Introduction to the Program and Review of Group Needs
9:15	Lecture: Providing for the Physical Needs of the Dying Person

10:00	Break
10:15	Lecture: Exploring the Social Dimensions for the Dying Person and His or Her Family
11:00	Lecture: Recognizing the Psychospiritual Needs of All
12:00	Lunch
12:30	Small Groups (Vignettes)
1:00	Large Group Discussion and Problem Solving
2:15	Wrap-up and Evaluation
2:30	Closure

REGISTRATION FORM

The Art of Caring for the Dying Person

April 20, 1998

Name:_____

Position/Title:_____

Work Area:_____

Shift:_____

Work Phone:_____

Other Phone:_____

Send to June McCall, Pastoral Services, or call extension 1234 for more information.

Workshop 5

When Someone Dies

WORKSHOP OBJECTIVES

In-service workshops provide an opportunity for participants to focus on principles and practices that provide for the quality care of our elderly.

This workshop focuses on the area of our common experiences of death and the effect it has on personal and professional living.

This workshop will help participants provide better health care for the aging through a better understanding of the aging and dying process, through self-assessment and reflection, and through designing treatment plans that reflect quality health care for the elderly.

SCHEDULE

9:00   Registration and Coffee

9:15   Attitudes About Death (Clips from the Media)

9:45   Lecture:
        Positive Dying in a Hospital? "The Power of Positive Dying."
        This presentation will focus on seemingly complex issues surrounding the concepts and experiences of death in a hospital setting.

10:45   Break

11:00   Life Plans: A Treatment Team Simulation
        "Good" death comes from positive life experiences. During this presentation, we will create a treatment plan for a typical resident, based on the assumption that the elderly person will die while in the hospital. The treatment plan will draw from resources of the various hospital disciplines.

12:30   Lunch

1:00   Lecture: A Caregiver's Experiences of Death and Positive Grief Responses
A funeral director will share his or her experiences and reflections as to how death and the grief process can be a more positive experience for those who are grieving.

2:30   Closure and Evaluation

CAREGIVER BELIEFS ABOUT ELDERCARE
IN A HOSPITAL/NURSING HOME

We are aware that it is difficult for an individual and for families to determine whether it is the right choice for a loved one to enter a hospital or nursing home.

- We believe we are here to help you.
- We believe each person has value.
- We believe that a caring and healthy community is important for each patient/resident.
- We believe that people live, learn, and grow throughout their lives.
- We believe that each of us makes daily choices.
- We believe it is important to talk about life, dying, and beliefs.
- We believe:
- We believe:
- We believe:

Workshop 6

Caring for the Caregiver

FLYER

Caring for the Caregiver

Day in and day out we provide loving
comfort to our residents, forming
relationships, extending ourselves, at
times, above and beyond what the job requires.

How and when do we care for ourselves?

Join us for an insightful
journey of exploring our strengths
and personal resources in developing
self-care skills.

May 29, 1998
9:00—11:00 a.m. Yellow Room
1:00—3:00 p.m. East Function Room
12:00—2:00 a.m. Yellow Room

Registration Requested—contact June at Pastoral Services, extension 1234.

FIGURE F. Being and Building a "Good Enough Caregiver"

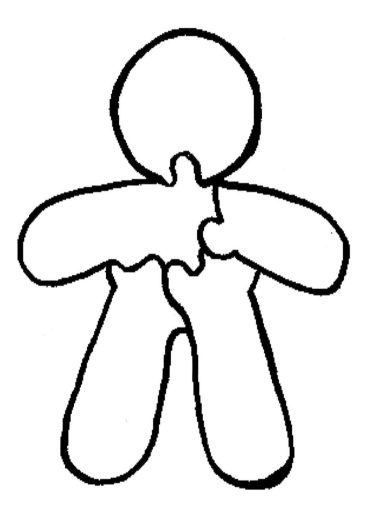

Introduction: Small groups brainstorm what elements make up a "good enough caregiver."

STAGES IN THE VOCATION OF A CAREGIVER

Stage One: Preparation to Be a Caregiver

This time is spent on preparing and learning to be a caregiver. The focus is on training and practice.

Stage Two: Entrance into Caregiving

The first few years in the vocational life of the caregiver are crucial to forming patterns of care and attitudes toward caregiving. Special emphasis needs to be placed on assisting and supporting caregivers during these early years.

Stage Three: Ongoing Caregiving

Throughout one's career, changes in focus, family, and sense of self are taking place. Services must be provided to caregivers in the midst of these processes of growth and change.

Stage Four: Exiting Caregiving

Exiting one's vocation may take place as the result of retirement, career change, or some crisis in the life or vocation of the caregiver or organization. Again, special needs must be addressed for this exit to be healthy for all concerned.

FIGURE G. Caregiver Goals and Needs

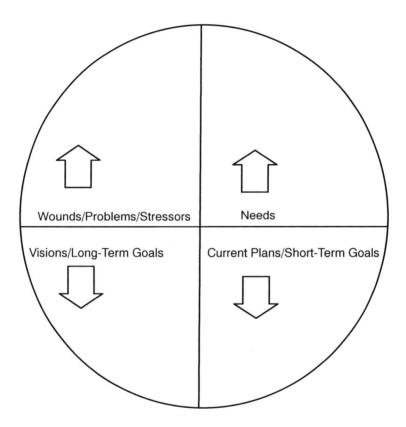

Instructions: This Circle is intended to help each individual caregiver reflect on his or her goals, problems (or wounds), needs, and vision (ideal) of self as caregiver.

Workshop 7

Brief In-Service Programs

SCHEDULE AND LECTURE TOPICS: TWO-HOUR MODEL

Grief and Loss

Introduction

Ask participants to introduce themselves and to include a couple of sentences about personal and/or professional issues that they are facing in the areas of death and dying, grief and loss. These responses are posted around the room to be included, when possible, in the rest of the program.

Death and Dying

- Stages of grief
- Dying person's expectations and wishes
- Discussion using participant's case material

Grief and Loss

- The grieving process
- Tasks of mourning
- Discussion using participant's case material

Closure

Evaluations

BEREAVEMENT LECTURE: TWENTY-MINUTE MODEL

General Observations

Mourning is:
- universal
- unique

- time limited
- process-oriented

Definitions

- Death and loss
- Bereavement
- Mourning
- Grief

Tasks of Mourning

- Accept the reality of loss
- Experience the pain of grief
- Detach and adjust to life without the deceased
- Reinvest energy in life and others

Phases of Mourning

- Shock and numbness
- Developing awareness and disorganization
- Reorganization
- Recovery

Brief Description of Phases

Bibliography

Abbott, John W. (Ed.) (1988). *Hospice Resource Manual for Local Churches.* New York: Pilgrim Press.

Arrington, Dawn and Karen Walborn (1989). "The Comfort Caregiver Concept." *Caring,* 8(12):24-27.

Balhorn, Ray and Ken Isaac (Prods.) (1995). *To Touch a Grieving Heart.* Healing ways to help ourselves and others walk the journey of grief. Salt Lake City, UT: Panacom Video.

Beck, Cornelia, Ruth Rawlins, and Sophronia Williams (1988). *Mental Health-Psychiatric Nursing, A Holistic Life Cycle Approach.* St. Louis: The C.V. Mosby Company.

Beland, Irene and Joyce Passos (1981). "Assessment of Spiritual Concerns." In *Clinical Nursing,* Fourth Edition, Beland and Passos (Eds.), 1237-1239. New York: Macmillan Publishing Company.

Benton, Richard G. (1978). *Death and Dying, Principles and Practices in Patient Care.* New York: D. VanNostrand Company.

Birren, James E. and R. Bruce Sloan (Ed.) (1980). *Handbook of Mental Health and Aging.* Englewood Cliffs, NJ: Prentice Hall, Inc.

Bonhoeffer, Dietrich (1986). *Meditating on the Word.* New York: Ballantine Books.

Bortz, Walter (1989). "Redefining Human Aging." *Journal of the American Geriatrics Society,* 37(11):1092-1096.

Bowlby, John (1980). *Attachment and Loss,* Volume Three, *Loss: Sadness and Depression.* New York: Basic Books, Inc.

Brim, Orville G. Jr., Howard E. Freeman, Sole Levine, and Norman A. Scotch (Eds.) (1970). *The Dying Patient.* New York: Russell Sage Foundation.

Buckman, Robert (1989). *I Don't Know What to Say, How to Help and Support Someone Who is Dying.* Boston: Little, Brown and Company.

Butler, Robert N. (1975). *Why Survive? Being Old in America.* New York: Harper & Row Publishers.

Caplan, Howard (1987). "It's Time We Helped Patients Die." *R.N.,* 50 (November):44-51.

Cassileth, Barrie R. and Peter A. Cassileth (1982). *Clinical Care of the Terminal Cancer Patient.* Philadelphia: Lea and Febiger.

Chekhov, Anton P. (1986). *The Schoolmistress and Other Stories.* Constance Garnett (Trans.). First published, 1886. New York: Ecco.

Clements, William (1980). "Pastoral Counseling." In *Counseling for the Growing Years: 65 and Over.* Charles Pulvino and Nicholas Colangelo (Eds.), 219-232. Minneapolis: Education Media Corp.

Crenshaw, David (1990). *Bereavement, Counseling the Grieving Throughout the Life Cycle.* New York: Continuum.

Cummings, Elaine and William Earl Henry (1961). *Growing Old: The Process of Disengagement.* New York: Basic Books.

Cutter, Fred (1974). *Coming to Terms with Death, How to Face the Inevitable with Wisdom and Dignity.* Chicago: Nelson-Hall Company.

DeMoss, Arthur and Nancy DeMoss (1974). *The Family Album.* Valley Forge, PA: The Family Album Publishers.

Doenges, Marilyn E., Mary C. Townsend, and Frances Moorhouse (1989). *Psychiatric Care Plans, Guidelines for Client Care.* Philadelphia: F.A. Davis Company.

Ebersole, Priscilla and Patricia Hess (1990). *Toward Healthy Aging, Human Needs and Nursing Response.* St. Louis: The C.V. Mosby Company.

Engel, George (1964). "Grief and Grieving." *American Journal of Nursing,* 64(9):93-98.

Erikson, Erik H. (1959/1963). *Childhood and Society.* New York: W.W. Norton and Company.

Erikson, Erik H. (1982). *The Life Cycle Completed.* New York: W.W. Norton and Company.

Flatt, Bill (1987). "Some Stages of Grief." *Journal of Religion and Health,* 26(2): 143-148.

Forbis, Patricia A. (1988). "Meeting Patients' Spiritual Needs." *Geriatric Nursing,* 9(3):158-159.

Fox, Tom (1989). "Borderline Personality Disorder: What Is Wrong with Them." Grand Rounds Presentation. Concord: New Hampshire Hospital, March 30.

Frankl, Viktor (1984). *Man's Search for Meaning.* New York: Pocket Books.

Freud, Sigmund (1956/1917). *Mourning and Melancholia, Standard Edition,* Volume Fourteen, James Strachey (Ed.). London: Hogarth Press.

Friedan, Betty (1993). *The Fountain of Age.* New York: Simon and Schuster.

Frost, Nicholas R. and Paula J. Clayton (1977). "Bereavement and Psychiatric Hospitalization." *Archives of General Psychiatry,* 34(10):1172-1175.

Garfield, Charles A. and Gary Jenkins (1981-1982). "Stress and Coping of Volunteers, Counseling the Dying and Bereaved." *Omega,* 12(1):1-13.

Gillick, Muriel R. (1989). "Long-Term Care Options for the Frail Elderly." *The Journal of the American Geriatrics Society,* 37(12): 1198-1203.

Glaser, Barney and Anselm L. Strauss (1968). *Time For Dying.* Chicago: Aldine Publishing Company.

Graham, Laurie (1990). *Rebuilding the House, One Woman's Passage Through Grief.* New York: Viking.

Green, Betty R. and Donald P. Irish (Eds.) (1971). *Death Education: Preparation for Living.* Cambridge, MA: Schenkman Publishing Company.

Gress, Lucille D. and Rose T. Bahr (1984). *The Aging Person, A Holistic Perspective.* St. Louis: The C.V. Mosby Company.

Guggenheim, Frederick and Myron F. Weiner (Eds.) (1984). *Manual of Psychiatric Consultation and Emergency Care.* New York: Jason Aronson, Inc.

Hall, Trish (1990). "Solace After Bereavement: Counseling Services Grow." *The New York Times,* May 20, 1990:1.

Hendricks, Jon and C. Davis Hendricks (1981). *Aging in Mass Society, Myths and Realities.* Cambridge, MA: Winthrop Publishers.

Hess, Beth B. and Elizabeth Markson (1980). *Aging and Old Age: An Introduction to Social Gerontology.* New York: Macmillan Publishing Company.

Holst, Lawrence E. (Ed.) (1985). *Hospital Ministry: The Role of the Chaplain Today.* New York: Crossroad.

Hommon, Donovan (1972). "An Assessment of the Effects of a Laboratory-Training Education Program in Bereavement Ministry Conducted by a Community Mental Health Center for Parish Clergymen." PhD dissertation. Boston: Boston University.

Horowitz, Mardi, Nancy Wilner, Charles Marmar, and Janice Krupnick (1980). "Pathological Grief and the Activation of Latent Self-Images." *American Journal of Psychiatry,* 137(10):1157-1162.

Hunter, Suzette (1992). "Adult Day Care: Promoting Quality of Life for the Elderly." *Journal of Gerontological Nursing,* 18(2):17-20.

Hurting, Wendy and Len Stwein (1990). "The Effect of Death Education and Experience on Nursing Students' Attitude Toward Death." *Journal of Advanced Nursing,* 15(1):29-34.

Jaeger, Dorthea and Leo W. Simmons (1970). *The Aged Ill, Coping with Problems in Geriatric Care.* New York: Appelton-Century-Crofts.

James, John W. and Frank Cherry (1988). *The Grief Recovery Handbook.* New York: Harper & Row Publishers.

Jordan, Merle R. (1986). *Taking on the Gods: The Task of the Pastoral Counselor.* Nashville: Abingdon Press.

Jung, Carl G. (1933). *Modern Man in Search of a Soul.* New York: Harcourt Brace Jovanovich, Inc.

Kübler-Ross, Elisabeth (1969). *On Death and Dying.* New York: Macmillan Publishing Company.

Kübler-Ross, Elisabeth (1975). *Death, The Final Stage of Hope.* Englewood Cliffs, NJ: Prentice Hall, Inc.

Kübler-Ross, Elisabeth and J. William Worden (1977-1978). "Attitudes of Death Workshop Attendees." *Omega,* 8(2):91-106.

Lapsley, James N. (1992). *Renewal in Late Life Through Pastoral Counseling.* New York: Paulist Press.

Lebow, Grace H. (1976). "Facilitating Adaptation in Anticipatory Mourning." *Social Casework,* 57(7):458-465.

Lego, Suzanne (Ed.) (1984). *The American Handbook of Psychiatric Nursing.* New York: J.B. Lippincott Company.

LeShan, Eda (1976). *Learning to Say Goodbye.* New York: Macmillan Publishing Company.

Leviton, Daniel (1971). The Role of Schools in Providing Death Education. In *Death Education: Preparation For Living.* Betty Green and Donald Irish (Eds.) Cambridge, MA: Schenkman Publishing Company.

Levy, Raymond and Felix Post (Eds.) (1982). *The Psychiatry of Later Life.* Oxford: Blackwell Scientific Publications.

Lewis, Clive Staples (1976). *A Grief Observed.* New York: Bantam Books.

Lindemann, Eric (1944). "Symptomatology and Management of Acute Grief." *American Journal of Psychiatry,* 101(2):141-148.

Maslow, Abraham (1954). *Motivation and Personality.* New York: Harper & Row Publishers.

Meyer, Charles (1987). "Eleven Myths About Death." *The Witness,* 3:6-10.

Mitchell, Kenneth R. and Herbert Anderson (1983). *All Our Losses, All Our Griefs, Resources for Pastoral Care.* Philadelphia: The Westminster Press.

Montapert, Alfred A. (1978). *The Way to Happiness, The Eternal Quest of Mankind.* Englewood Cliffs, NJ: Prentice Hall Inc.

Murrell, Stanley and Samuel Himmelfarb (1989). "Effects of Attachment Bereavement and Pre-Event Conditions on Subsequent Depressive Symptoms in Older Adults." *Psychology and Aging,* 4(2):166-172.

Mussen, Paul Henry, John Conger, Jerome Kagan, and James Geiwitz (1979). *Psychological Development: A Life Span Approach.* New York: Harper & Row Publishers.

New Hampshire Hospital Policy and Procedures Manual (1997). New Hampshire Hospital, Concord, New Hampshire.

Niebuhr, H. Richard (1989). *Faith on Earth: An Inquiry into the Structure of Human Faith.* New Haven, CT: Yale University Press.

Norberg, Astrid and Kenneth Asplund (1990). "Caregivers Experience of Caring for Severely Demented Patients." *Western Journal of Nursing Research,* 12(1):75-84.

Nouwen, Henri J. (1979). *The Wounded Healer, Ministry in Contemporary Society.* New York: Doubleday.

Oates, Wayne E. (1978). *The Religious Care of the Psychiatric Patient.* Philadelphia: The Westminster Press.

Oliver, David B. and Sally Tureman (1988). *The Human Factor in Nursing Home Care.* Binghamton, NY: The Haworth Press.

Oswald, Roy M. (1991). *Clergy Self-Care, Finding A Balance for Effective Ministry.* Trinity Church, New York City, The Alban Institute.

Parke-Davis (Sponsor) (1994). *Caring for the Caregiver: A Guide to Living with Alzheimer's Disease.* Morris Plains, NJ: Warner-Lambert Company.

Parkes, Colin Murray (1964). "Recent Bereavement as a Cause of Mental Illness." *British Journal of Psychiatry,* 110(465):198-204.

Parkes, Colin Murray (1972). *Bereavement: Studies of Grief in Adult Life.* New York: International University Press.

Parkes, Colin Murray (1979). *Bereavement: Studies of Grief in Adult Life.* New York: International University Press, Inc.

Parkes, Colin Murray and Robert Stuart Weis (1983). *Recovery from Bereavement.* New York: Basic Books.

Peterson, Elisabeth (1987). "How to Meet Your Client's Spiritual Needs." *Journal of Psychosocial Nursing,* 25(5):34-39.

Prucho, R. A. and S. L. Potashnik (1989). "Caregiving Spouses: Physical and Mental Health Perspective." *The Journal of the American Geriatric Society,* 37:697-705.

Pulvino, Charles J. and Nicholas Colanoelo (Eds.) (1980). *Counseling for the Growing Years: 65 and Over.* Minneapolis: Educational Media Corporation.

Pumphrey, Rev. John A. (1997). "Recognizing Your Patient's Spiritual Needs." *Nursing,* 7(12):64-70.

Ramshaw, Elaine (1987). *Ritual and Pastoral Care.* Philadelphia: Fortress Press.

Rando, Therese (1984). *Grief, Dying and Death, Clinical Interventions for Caregivers.* Champaign, IL: Research Press Company.

Raphael, Beverly (1983). *The Anatomy of Bereavement.* New York: Basic Books.

Rathbone-McCuan, Eloise and Joan Hishimi (1982). *Isolated Elders, Health and Social Intervention.* Rockville, MD: Aspen Systems Corporation.

Rawlins, Ruth and Patricia Heacock (1988). *Clinical Manual of Psychiatric Nursing.* St. Louis: The C.V. Mosby Company.

Reich, John W., Alex J. Zautra, and Charles A. Guarnaccia (1989). "Effects of Disability and Bereavement on the Mental Health and Recovery of Older Adults." *Psychology and Aging,* 4(1):57-59.

Sanders, Catherine M. (1989). *Grief: The Mourning After, Dealing with Adult Bereavement.* New York: John Wiley and Sons, Inc.

Schoenberg, Bernard et al. (Eds.) (1979). *Loss and Grief: Psychological Management in Medical Practice.* New York: Columbia University Press.

Schreck, Nancy and Maureen Leach (1986). *Psalms Anew: In Inclusive Language.* Winona, MN: Saint Mary's Press.

Schreiber, LeAnn (1990). *Midstream: The Story of a Mother's Death and a Daughter's Renewal.* New York: Viking.

Seaman, Lennie and Leonard Roth (1989). "Active Treatment for Long-Term Care Psychiatric Patients." *Geriatric Nursing,* 10(5):232-234.

Sevensky, Robert L. (1982). "The Religious Physician." *Journal of Religion and Health,* 21(3):254-263.

Shelly, Judith Allen, Sandra D. John, Arlene Miller, Arlynne Ostlund, Verna J. Carson, Mertie Potter, Kenneth L. Williams, Sidney Whitney Langston, Mary Berg, and Barbara Nelson (1983). *Spiritual Dimensions of Mental Health.* Downers Grove, IL: InterVarsity Press.

Shulman, Kenneth I. (1978). "Suicide and Parasuicide in Old Age: A Review." *Age and Aging,* 7: 201-209.

Smithson, June (1987). "Death and Dying. How Do You Cope? How Should You Cope?" *O.T. Advance,* 3(8):3-6.

Solzhenitsyn, Alexander (1968). *Cancer Ward.* New York: Bantam Books.

Stone, Howard W. (1996). "Grief Ministry in Transition." *The Journal of Pastoral Care,* Fall, 50(3):269-273.

Stroebe, Wolfgang and Margaret Stroebe (1987). *Bereavement and Health.* Cambridge, MA: Cambridge University Press.

Sullender, R. Scott (1981). "Saint Paul's Approach to Grief: Clarifying the Ambiguity." *Journal of Religion and Health,* 20(1): 63-74.

Tanner, Ira J. (1976). *Healing the Pain of Everyday Loss.* Minneapolis: Windsor Press, Inc.

Temes, Robert (1984). *Living with an Empty Chair, A Guide Through Grief.* New York: New Horizon Press.

Thomas, William H. (1996). *Life Worth Living, How Someone You Love Can Still Enjoy Life in a Nursing Home.* Acton, MA: VanderWyk and Burnham.

Walrond-Skinner, Sue (1986). *A Dictionary of Psychotherapy.* New York: Routledge and Kegan Paul.

Ward, Russell A. (1979). *The Aging Experience: An Introduction to Social Gerontology.* New York: J.B. Lippincott Company.

Weisman, Avery D. (1972). *On Dying and Denying: A Psychiatric Study of Terminality.* New York: Behavioral Publications, Inc.

Weiss, Jules C. (1984). *Expressive Therapy with Elders and the Disabled.* Binghamton, NY: The Haworth Press.

Westburg, Granger E. (1961). *Good Grief.* Philadelphia: Fortress Press.

White House Conference on Aging (1971). *Spiritual Well-Being.* Washington DC: US Government Printing Office.

Williams, Robert (Ed.) (1973). *To Live and To Die: When, Why, and How.* New York: Springer-Verlag.

Worden, J. William (1982). *Grief Counseling and Grief Therapy: A Handbook for the Mental Health Practitioner.* New York: Springer Publishing Company.

Worden, J. William and William Proctor (1976). *PDA—Breaking Free of Fear to Live a Better Life Now.* (Personal Death Awareness.) Englewood Cliffs, NJ: Prentice Hall Inc.

Yalom, Irvin D. and Sophia Vinogradow (1988). "Bereavement Groups: Techniques and Themes." *International Journal of Group Psychotherapy,* 38(4):419-445.

Young, John L. and Ezra E. H. Griffith (1989). "The Development and Practice of Pastoral Counseling." *Hospital and Community Psychiatry,* 40(3):271-276.

Index

Page numbers followed by the letter "f" indicate figures.

Order Your Own Copy of
This Important Book for Your Personal Library!

GRIEF EDUCATION FOR CAREGIVERS OF THE ELDERLY

_____ in hardbound at $29.95 (ISBN: 0-7890-0498-4)

COST OF BOOKS_____

OUTSIDE USA/CANADA/
MEXICO: ADD 20%_____

POSTAGE & HANDLING_____
(US: $3.00 for first book & $1.25
for each additional book)
Outside US: $4.75 for first book
& $1.75 for each additional book)

SUBTOTAL_____

IN CANADA: ADD 7% GST_____

STATE TAX_____
(NY, OH & MN residents, please
add appropriate local sales tax)

FINAL TOTAL_____
(If paying in Canadian funds,
convert using the current
exchange rate. UNESCO
coupons welcome.)

☐ **BILL ME LATER:** ($5 service charge will be added)
(Bill-me option is good on US/Canada/Mexico orders only;
not good to jobbers, wholesalers, or subscription agencies.)

☐ Check here if billing address is different from
shipping address and attach purchase order and
billing address information.

Signature_____

☐ **PAYMENT ENCLOSED: $**_____

☐ **PLEASE CHARGE TO MY CREDIT CARD.**

☐ Visa   ☐ MasterCard   ☐ AmEx   ☐ Discover
☐ Diners Club
Account # _____

Exp. Date _____

Signature _____

Prices in US dollars and subject to change without notice.

NAME _____

INSTITUTION _____

ADDRESS _____

CITY _____

STATE/ZIP _____

COUNTRY _____ COUNTY (NY residents only) _____

TEL _____ FAX _____

E-MAIL_____
May we use your e-mail address for confirmations and other types of information? ☐ Yes   ☐ No

Order From Your Local Bookstore or Directly From
The Haworth Press, Inc.
10 Alice Street, Binghamton, New York 13904-1580 • USA
TELEPHONE: 1-800-HAWORTH (1-800-429-6784) / Outside US/Canada: (607) 722-5857
FAX: 1-800-895-0582 / Outside US/Canada: (607) 772-6362
E-mail: getinfo@haworthpressinc.com
PLEASE PHOTOCOPY THIS FORM FOR YOUR PERSONAL USE.